Meanderings in Medical History

Book Four

Meanderings in Medical History

Book Four

MICHAEL NEVINS

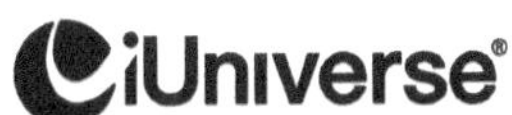

MEANDERINGS IN MEDICAL HISTORY BOOK FOUR

iUniverse books may be ordered through booksellers or by contacting:

iUniverse
1663 Liberty Drive
Bloomington, IN 47403
www.iuniverse.com
1-800-Authors (1-800-288-4677)

ISBN: 978-1-5320-1260-0 (sc)
ISBN: 978-1-5320-1261-7 (e)

Print information available on the last page.

iUniverse rev. date: 12/12/2016

INTRODUCTION

When I began a two year term as president of the Medical History Society of New Jersey in 2011, I thought that it would be fun to gather in one place several things I'd written in the past that pertained to my home state's medical history. The result was *Meanderings in New Jersey's Medical History* which contained twenty-two essays whose only unifying theme was that they had something to do with The Garden State. Having completed that project, there were many more subjects unrelated to New Jersey that had interested me over the years so a second book soon followed that I called *More Meanderings in Medical History*. Indeed there was so much material that the next year came *Still More Meanderings in Medical History* and by then I was sure that this had satisfied my compulsion to write - but not quite. During the next two years new subjects attracted my interest so that with this latest volume the trilogy has expanded to a quartet and, dispensing with adjectives, this one is simply titled *Meanderings in Medical History: Book Four.*

I have no illusions that these unrelated and unreferenced studies are worthy of a scholarly thesis; rather, they were written merely to amuse myself and if others share my interests, all the better. But "meandering" does seem an appropriate verb to describe my approach for, as should be evident from perusing the range of chapter headings in these books (see following), my taste is eclectic. Inspiration for many chapters came from unexpected experiences - such as a casual conversation, a museum visit or a perplexing roadside historical marker. With rare repetitions or overlaps, each chapter is free-standing and can be read in any sequence. And if that seems confusing, it should be understood that for a time each subject interested me enough to prompt exploration and writing my findings down provided a way of coming to closure and allowing me to move on to something else. So without further explanation, what follows are seventeen more meanderings in medical history, bringing total chapters in the four books to seventy-eight.

CONTENTS

PREVIOUS MEANDERINGS.

BOOK ONE: ***Meanderings in New Jersey's Medical History***

1. "A Very Healthful Air"
2. Hackensack's First Hospital: October-November, 1776
3. You've Got Mail
4. The Stormy Petrel of American Medical Education
5. From Brandy to Graham Crackers
6. A Country Doctor Calls For Help
7. Essex County Doctors Go To War
8. Doctor, Lawyer, Indian Chief - and Poet
9. *Le Medcin Malgre Lui*
10. The Old Doctor's Garden
11. Treating the Sun Starved
12. Spectrochrome Therapy
13. The Perils of Pus
14. A Caring Physician
15. Abraham Flexner: The Princeton Years
16. Newark's Polio Panics
17. Disaster at Bari
18. Dr. Evil
19. Dr. X
20. A Right to Die: The Sad Story of Karen Ann Quinlan
21. When Is Enough Enough?
22. Shooting the Messenger Twelve Years After He's Dead

BOOK TWO: ***More Meanderings in Medical History***

1. All Fall Down
2. An Eponymic Clash
3. La Salpetriere
4. Medical Cut Ups
5. The Autocrat and the Apostle
6. Bad Seeds
7. A Duty To Die
8. Honorary Paternity
9. Flexner's Report

BOOK THREE: ***Still More Meanderings in Medical History***

1. A FACE IN THE CROWD

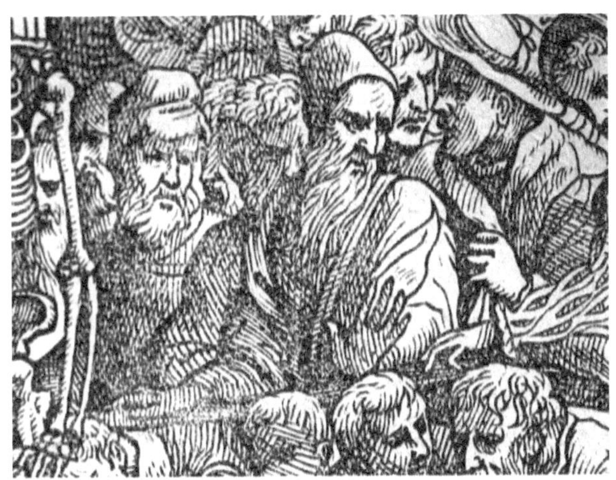

A friend of mine Dr. Jeffrey Levine for many years has been fascinated by minute visual details contained in the 16th century anatomic atlas familiarly known as the Fabrica that was produced by Andreas Vesalius. He once suggested to me that an obscure background figure seen on the book's illustrated title page may have been a Jewish friend of Vesalius and, intrigued by this possibility, I decided to investigate. What follows here is adapted from a talk given by Dr. Levine and me in 2014 at the New York Academy of Medicine on the occasion of the 500th anniversary of Vesalius' birth. (The full article was published in KOROT: The Israel Journal of the History of Medicine and Science. vol. 23 (2015-2016) 237-256)

The world literature is voluminous concerning Andreas Vesalius' iconic *De humani corporis fabrica* (On The Structure of the Human Body) which was published in 1543. As James Ball wrote in 1910, "Vesalius overthrew the idol of authority in anatomy and taught us to look at Nature with our own eye." Harvey Cushing, one of the Flemish anatomist's most enthusiastic biographers, observed that no book has ever received such acclaim yet was read by so few." In our own time fewer still have seen more than a reproduction or two of a skeleton or "muscleman" in a history book.

The massive atlas, known as the *Fabrica*, contains 659 folio pages of text, 34 pages of index and 6 pages of preface, but its importance relates to the 273 graphics themselves. Scholarly attention has focused mainly on those aspects relating to the *Fabrica's* seminal role in medical history but the elaborate title page is of particular beauty -- as historian Charles D. O'Malley said of it, "there can be no question that the woodcut ranks among the finest achievements of the art of the engraver in the 16th century." Vesalius is shown performing a public dissection upon a female cadaver in an anatomic theater, surrounded by a motley crowd of ninety onlookers. Since in the accompanying text Vesalius didn't identify any of them, historians have had a field day speculating about individual identities, picking over fine details as assiduously as the Flemish anatomist examined muscles and bones.

Vesalius was known to personally plan every detail so there was nothing haphazard about the mob scene displayed on the title page where perhaps hidden in plain sight were background features which reflected conditions in 16th century Europe. If deliberately placed by Vesalius, there were numerous precedents for including coded content in Renaissance art. Indeed Benjamin Blech and Roy Doliner suggested in *The Sistine Secrets* that Michelangelo's ceiling in the Sistine Chapel, painted some three decades earlier (1508-1512), contained subversive symbols of which the artist's patron Pope Julius II wouldn't have approved. The authors noted that "every single element of Renaissance art has an inner significance: the choice of subject and protagonists, the faces selected for different characters in the work…their positions, stances, gestures and juxtapositions…all have hidden meanings."

Appearing in the top row of the dissection scene is a bearded man wearing a cylindrical hat - a single face in the motley crowd jostling to have a look. He is removed from the main action and appears troubled either by what he is witnessing or by what his neighbor is whispering in his ear. Over the centuries, scholars have suggested that he was Lazarus de Frigeis (alt. Lazarro Hebraeo Frigeis, Lazari Ebreo, Lazaro Freschi) a Jewish physician whom Vesalius wrote had taught him the Hebrew words for certain bones. In medieval paintings Jews often were depicted as goats, dogs, monkeys or odious characters but this individual appears among the others as an equal and wears no distinguishing badges to mark him as a Jew. However, the University of Padua where Vesalius was working was a center of Humanism where Jewish students were exempted from wearing distinctive hats or badges; on occasion, privileged Jewish physicians also were granted this concession. Indeed, both in appearance and garb this figure is almost identical with a woodcut engraving of a contemporary Jewish physician Moses Hamon (1496-1554) whose family fled Spain for Constantinople and who in his maturity became personal physician to Sultan Suleiman the Magnificent.

Perhaps placing Lazarus de Frigeis in the crowd around the dissection table was a way of expressing gratitude for his help with Hebrew and in the accompanying text Vesalius provided additional information. According to Charles O'Malley's translation of Vesalius' Latin:

> *Almost all [of the lettering] was taken from the Hebrew translations of Avicenna through the efforts of Lazaro de Frigeis, a distinguished Jewish physician and close friend with whom I have been accustomed to translate Avicena.*

Historian Daniel Garrison's translation (2013) was almost identical:

> *Almost all taken from a Hebrew translation of Avicenna with the aid of a prominent physician and close friend of mine, Lazarus Hebraeus de Frigeis with whom I am accustomed to work on Avicenna.*

It wasn't Vesalius' practice to publicly acknowledge either friends or foes so such generous recognition is noteworthy, especially when referring to a Jew. According to historian Jonathan Elukin, though, it's simplistic to view Jewish life merely in terms of persecution and marginalization for although conditions during the 15th and 16th centuries may have been harsh, many Jews developed social relationships with gentiles and there was a network of Christian, Jewish and Muslim intellectuals which spanned the Mediterranean world. Nevertheless if friendship between Vesalius and Lazarus de Frigeis in relatively tolerant Padua would not have been remarkable, surely it might have been risky during this tempestuous period.

By the 1540s Jews had long since been expelled from Iberia, France and most of Europe. In Italy there'd been an influx of émigrés and there were established ghettoes in Venice (1516) and later Florence and Rome. However, far more concern was directed toward Protestant reformers in northern Europe than with downtrodden Jews. To be sure, with the onset of the Renaissance many of Italy's elite were seeking Jewish scholars for personal instruction in Hebrew. Humanists not only returned to Greek but also to Hebrew and by 1514 Hebrew was a required subject at the Vatican university.

At best, Vesalius' knowledge of Hebrew was rudimentary so in order to provide Hebrew words for bones he needed help. Although his "close" friend Lazarus (an alternate translation describes him as his "intimate" friend) may have taught him Hebrew equivalents, modern scholars have suggested that the result was "most chaotic and variable. To be sure Hebrew words appeared in only three pages and one marginal note in the massive *Fabrica* suggesting that Hebrew medical terminology was not yet standardized during the Vesalian period.

During the Middle Ages Avicenna's fourteen volume *Canon of Medicine* was a standard medical text at many universities, but by the early 16th century some iconoclasts were complaining about the "tyranny" of Avicenna who to them represented the stultified Arabic influence which then "occupied" Italian medical schools. Nevertheless, the young Flemish anatomist's departure from Galenic hegemony angered his conservative elders. Avicenna surely represented an important virtual ally for when there was a conflict between Galen and Aristotle, especially about anatomy, Avicenna often took the side of the latter, which supported Vesalius' contention that Galen was not infallible.

A Hebrew translation of the *Canon* which appeared in Naples in 1491 seems to have been the text used by Vesalius and Lazarus and soon several more Hebrew translations were published in Venice. One was written by the prominent Jewish physician Jacob Mantino, a contemporary of Vesalius, who reputedly was the most prolific translator of Greek and Arabic medical texts to Hebrew. Mantino's family had been exiled from Spain in 1492 and by the time he arrived in Venice in 1528, as an eminent physician he was exempted from wearing the pointed "Jew hat." Jacob Mantino came to the attention of Pope Paul III who employed him as a court physician and later appointed him professor of medicine at the University of Rome (using the name Giacomo Ebreo). But the life of a court physician could be perilous and Mantino ran afoul of Cardinal Sadolet who denounced him and convinced the Pope to issue a Bull which temporarily suspended the privileges of all Jewish physicians. There can be no doubt that both Vesalius and Lazarus were well aware of the shifting fortunes of Jewish physicians like Jacob Mantino and, as we shall soon see, this might have been influential in events to come.

WHO WAS LAZARUS DE FRIGEIS?

Although the authoritative biographer Charles O'Malley stated that our bearded spectator in the *Fabrica's* dissection scene "most likely" was Vesalius' Jewish friend, further identification of him remained "an unsolved puzzle." During the 16th century Jews didn't use surnames and Frigeis probably referred to a location, probably in northern Europe - Lazarus from Frigeis. Historian Mordecai Etziony was critical of the Hebrew writing used in the *Fabrica*: "If...we are to suppose that both the Hebrew equivalents and their transliterations were written for Vesalius by his Hebrew friend Lazarus de Frigeis...then we must credit the latter with little knowledge of Hebrew since some of the grammatical mistakes are inexcusable for a connoisseur of the language."

Whatever his aptitude in Hebrew, several modern Italian scholars have suggested that at the very same time that the two friends were studying Avicenna, Lazarus had more important things on his mind. Indeed he was in the process of becoming a New Christian or *converso* and after his conversion, probably in 1550, changed his name to Giovanni Battista de' Freschi Olivi. What follows next is derived from several Italian sources which, in turn, were based on published records of the Venetian Inquisition which was heating up during the 1540s.

There being no evidence that Lazarus de Frigeis was either a "distinguished" or "prominent" physician, It is difficult to understand why Vesalius referred to his friend in this way. Indeed it would seem that the sobriquet might more aptly be applied to his own physician father Raphael de Phrigiis (a.k.a. Raffaele Fritschke) who not only was a scholar but also an influential rabbi in Padua and an authority on Jewish law. When Raphael died in 1540, his will requested a traditional Ashkenazic Jewish burial and left a considerable fortune to his three sons Lazarus, Benjamin and Isaac. However, his extensive collection of books on humanities, logic, medicine, philosophy and Hebrew were bequeathed to Lazarus alone. Apparently he was the most studious son and it's possible that the Hebrew translation of Avicenna's *Canon* that the friends were reading came from Raphael's library.

After Lazarus completed his medical studies in Padua in August 1540, he was granted permission to take the examination which would qualify him to practice medicine in Padua, including care of Christian patients. Vesalius had obtained his medical diploma in 1539 and immediately the Flemish prodigy was appointed chief of surgery – an impressive fast track. Since Lazarus didn't graduate until the next year he was a novice so that the relationship between these "close friends" must have been more like that of teacher and student, albeit they probably were about the same age.

In 1547, five years after the manuscript of the *Fabrica* was finished, Lazarus moved to Venice where he joined the Ashkenazic community and petitioned the chief rabbi for permission to live in the "old" ghetto. (In fact this was a misnomer because the "old" *ghetto vecchio* was an expansion in 1541 of the original *ghetto nuovo* of 1516 in order to accommodate an influx of Levantine (Turkish) Jews.) It's unclear why Lazarus wished to live in this area which was described as being "old, ruined and in a bad state" but by 1550, shortly after the time of his conversion, as Giovanni he was living outside the ghetto and by the next year he was granted additional privileges that were afforded Christian physicians.

In his new identity Giovanni became a virulent Jew-hater and participated in a Venetian commission which one Sabbath day (October 21, 1553) burned more than a thousand copies of the Talmud and other holy books in the Piazza San Marco. His singular contribution was to advise the commission on what blasphemous books in addition to the Babylonian and Jerusalem Talmuds should be heaped on the fire. The former Lazarus de Frigeis boasted, "I have persecuted, and continue to persecute, those blasphemies and insults that are contained in the books of the Jews, and will go on so doing as long as I live, and after death if that is possible, taking no account of danger, enmity, retaliation or injuries to my body."

Whether Lazaro/Giovanni's appalling behavior was sincere or a way of covering his tracks is pure speculation but the *converso* didn't get off easily. He'd convinced his elderly mother Elena to be baptized along with the rest of the family (when his wife refused he divorced her) but although she agreed Elena had grave misgivings. She became deranged and an accuser claimed that at Sunday Mass "she made ugly faces, said bad words" and yelled at the priest, "You're lying through your teeth." In 1555 the matter was formally investigated by The Holy Office of Venice which concluded that the old woman's ravings were due to madness rather than the words of a deliberate blasphemer. During his mother's trial, testimony given by a woman named Maddalena identified Giovanni as the former Jewish physician Lazarus, but now he had some standing with the Holy Office since he'd collaborated in the destruction of the Talmud. Giovanni argued that his mother was possessed by evil spirits and either was a lunatic or melancholic; surely this was the work of the Devil singling out the mother of a fearless prosecutor of Jewish blasphemy. Perhaps because of his stellar record, when no public institution would take her in, Elena was committed to perpetual confinement in her son's house. When Lazarus died, sometime between 1555 and 1560, presumably he was not buried alongside his father because the Jewish community considered him to be a turncoat – a hostile enemy of his people.

PADUA: 1537--1542

Even before Lazarus' conversion, a social bond between these two Paduan physicians would have been perfectly natural since the university was notable for its tolerance of Jewish students and faculty members. Despite its proximity to the Vatican, Padua was part of the free Venetian state and was located some twenty-five miles south of the port city. Humanists believed that a person's worth should be judged by their breadth of knowledge and culture, by accomplishments and not by fortune or religion, and the University of Padua sought out the best teachers regardless of their personal beliefs. It relaxed the requirement that graduates avow their belief in Christianity as a prerequisite to obtaining a degree. The first Jewish medical student graduated in 1409 and was followed by hundreds more from all over Europe – eighty between 1517 and 1619. Indeed there were several Jewish faculty members besides Lazarus during this period, including the esteemed Elijah Delmedigo.

The years that Vesalius spent in Padua corresponded with his first public questioning of Galen's accuracy and it was there that he worked on the *Tabulae Anatomicae* (1538), the *Fabrica* (1543) and the abridged manual called the *Epitome* that was published the same month. When the woodcuts of the *Fabrica* were finished, probably in Venice in August 1542 after about three years of work, Vesalius took almost a year off to accompany his precious treasures to Basel where for some seven months he supervised the atlas's completion by the accomplished printer Johannes Oporinus.

1543: A MOMENTOUS YEAR

Another epic work of science which appeared in 1543 was Copernicus' *De revolutionibus orbium celestium.* (Legend has it that Copernicus first saw his great work completed on the very last day of his life when he died of a stroke.) That same year Charles V united with England's Henry VIII and attacked France, but more pertinent to Vesalius' future were three other events which occurred at about this time. One was that Charles V appointed his sixteen year old son Philip as the regent of Spain, who a dozen years later when his father abdicated would assume most of his father's mantles. (Charles had some 79 titles and once complained that they were "more than one head can carry.") Philip was more religiously orthodox and stiff-necked than his father and under his leadership Spain would become the center of the Counter-Reformation. At about this same time the zealous Cardinal Gian Pietro Caraffa initiated the Inquisition in Rome modeled on the Spanish precedent. Six years earlier his baleful influence had been felt in Venice when Caraffa served as a papal agent and now he vowed "to suppress and uproot, permitting no trace [of heresy] to remain… even if my own father were a heretic, I would gather the wood to burn him." Books were prohibited from being published without approval of his Holy Office and liberalizing doctrines established by the Council of Trent were suspended. Considering all this, it's conceivable that Lazarus de Frigeis' post conversion cooperation with the Inquisition may have been prompted by prevailing suspicion of the faithfulness of *conversos,* burning Jewish books serving as evidence of his sincerity. 1543 also was the year that Martin Luther published his virulently anti-Semitic treatise *The Jews and Their Lies* so that at the same time that Vesalius published his epic work and joined the imperial court as personal physician of Charles V, Europe was in the midst of political and religious turmoil. Surely his choice of what to say or not say in the next edition of the *Fabrica* must be understood within this context.

THE VENETIAN INQUISITION

Just what was the political and religious context in the Republic of Venice which governed Padua during Vesalius' most productive years? As described by Brian Pullan, Venice served as a transit town for people on a spiritual journey between two faiths and on a physical voyage between the monolithically Catholic states of western Europe and the religious pluralism of the Ottoman lands.

> *Unambiguously Catholic but famed for its "liberty", it sheltered believer and unbeliever, atheist and zealot, the hesitant and the convinced.... It was often in Venice that Europeans of Jewish blood made their final choice between Christianity and Judaism; those who hesitated and faced both ways, neither conforming fully nor vowing themselves permanently to either creed, were most likely to suffer at the Inquisition's hands."*

By 1540 an Inquisition was functioning in Venice consisting of a papal nuncio, the patriarch and a Franciscan inquisitor. In 1542 Pope Paul III revived the Inquisition in Rome and by 1547 things began to heat up in Venice. That was four years after Vesalius left to join the imperial court, but a climate of distrust had been building for years. Although professing Jews and people of Jewish descent were seldom a preoccupation of the Inquisitors, they were an alien community and individual cases heard by the Tribunals involved any form of heresy, apostasy or blasphemy – such as the trial of Elena de' Freschi Olivi.

When Cardinal Caraffa was elected Pope Paul IV in 1555, religious fanaticism and persecution heightened. Now Jews, who had been expelled from southern Italy (The Kingdom of Naples) during the 1530s and had found safe haven in Ancona, were given their choice of two options: baptism or burning – sixty three chose the former, twenty four the latter while others fled for their lives· According to historian Sheila Hale:

> *Under Paul IV the creativity and search for the truth that we think of as hallmarks of the Italian Renaissance were temporarily replaced by suppression, blind orthodoxy and fear of innovation; but only for as long as he lived. Paul's death four years after his election was greeted in Rome with jubilation. Mobs rampaged through the streets toppling statues of the late unlamented pope and smashing open the cells in which prisoners of the inquisition had been incarcerated. He was succeeded by the moderate conventionally religious Pius IV, an affable*

man and able bureaucrat, who immediately pardoned those who had participated in the riots and went on to revive the Council of Trent.

There was constant tension between the Roman and Venetian Inquisitions, the latter being less doctrinaire and intended mainly to reconcile religious duty with political independence and economic interest. Its more practical spirit was closer to that of the court of Charles V, the most powerful ruler in Europe, with whom Vesalius's career now would be linked.

THE SECOND EDITION

When Vesalius returned to Padua from Basel after publishing his *magnum opus*, he found that the mood had changed. Rivals had emerged at the university and most hurtful of all was his former Parisian mentor Jacobus Sylvius who publicly called him a "madman…whose pestilential breath poisons Europe." Vesalius resigned his teaching position and accepted an offer to become physician to Charles V. To be sure, it may have been his intention all along for he'd dedicated his *Fabrica* "To the Divine Charles V, The mightiest and most unvanquished Emperor" and perhaps these obsequious words helped gain him a place in the Imperial court. Of course it didn't hurt that his father had served as the Emperor's personal apothecary. (The *Epitome* published the same month as the *Fabrica* was dedicated to Prince Phillip of Spain.) In this stricter environment it would have been prudent for the wary Vesalius to temper any overt signs of admiration for a Jewish doctor in the next edition of his *Fabrica*.

It is unclear why Vesalius felt the need to produce an updated version of the *Fabrica*. Naturally he wished to make corrections and improvements but apparently there also was some disagreement about timing with his printer Oporinus favoring waiting until more of the first edition was sold. When the second edition appeared in 1555 its title page had been done over, the craftsmanship quite different and clearly the hand of an inferior artist. O'Malley suggested that the original wood block may have been damaged since it was used not only for the *Fabrica* but also for the *Epitome* which was printed at virtually the same time. Whatever the reason the revised title page contained several intriguing modifications.

In the second edition Vesalius' head and garments appear markedly different, expressions on many of the gawking faces have changed and, perhaps as a concession to the Inquisitors, now the genitals of the corpse are obscured and a nude figure has been clothed. Also there are ominous hints of double meanings – the magisterial staff originally clutched by the skeleton has transformed into a scythe and now the border around the dedication shield is wrapped in ropes and chains. Does the sudden appearance of a ram in the foreground refer symbolically to a familiar medieval iconographic reference to Satan? Or to a scapegoat? It appears as if these newly added images are indicators of deadlier times.

Of course production of such a massive undertaking as the *Fabrica* had to be a joint effort involving anatomist, artist, woodcarver and printer. It was customary for the draughtsman to place the design on wood blocks; then highly skilled craftsmen would cut away the wood to leave the drawn lines projecting in relief. Vesalius was a perfectionist and, no doubt, supervised every phase of the production. The current consensus is that the engraved frontispiece of the first *Fabrica* as well as the portrait of Vesalius probably were done by his countryman Jan Stefan van Kalkar (Calcar) who had joined Titian's Venetian studio in 1536 and had done three drawings for Vesalius's earlier *Tabulae Anatomicae*. However there have been many dissenters. Professor O'Malley doubted that Kalkar was the primary artist and suggested that TItian himself at least may have consulted on design because of the superb artistry of the first *Fabrica*. Vesalius complained of the enormous financial expense incurred to induce skilled artists to undertake the unpleasant, odoriferous work and the need for him to direct "the eye, hand and the intelligence" of the artist(s). He also remarked on their "obstinacy" and sarcastically considered himself more unfortunate than the criminal whose body he'd been dissecting. All of this suggests that there were more than one artist, but regardless of who illustrated the first edition, even less is known about who did the title page for the second edition. Markedly inferior in technique, it is evident that it was done by the hand of a far less talented artist -- and certainly *not* by Kalcar who had died in the interim in 1547 at age 48.

In the 1555 version of the *Fabrica* the figure of Lazarus remains in place, albeit looking rather wild-eyed and, for an unknown reason, now his previously raised left hand is hidden from view. Perhaps these were deliberate changes or, more likely, reflected the technique of a different artist. But most important for our purpose is that now in the accompanying text when describing Lazarus de Frigeis, Vesalius dropped the phrase "distinguished Jewish physician" referring to him only as his close friend. (Noted by O'Malley and confirmed by Garrison.) Daring to criticize the immortal Galen was bold enough and perhaps to include anything which might be interpreted as Judaizing could be catastrophic. O'Malley suggested that "improvements" in the 1555 text were intended to get rid of many redundancies, including omission of comments on his personal life and that of his friends. Perhaps so, but as Nutton observed, in the second edition Vesalius removed references to "purposes of the Creator… [which] may hint at the growing religious intolerance at the Imperial court that made problematic any theological utterances unless ecclesiastically sanctioned."

In a letter written to a friend in 1546, Vesalius described how after joining the imperial court, he reacted to criticism by burning his own books:

> *When I left Italy to apply myself to the court [of Charles V]…I burned everything, with the intention of restraining myself somewhat in writing. However, I have often regretted the upsurge and have felt sorry for not listening to the advice of my friends, who were present. Although, as far as the notes are concerned, I am very much pleased, because even if they would still be in my possession I would not feel tempted to publish them, as I can easily foresee that they would make each and every one my enemy…I have since repented more than once of my impatience, and regretted that I did not take the advice of the friends who were then with me.*

Stephen Joffe suggests that this impetuous gesture was "the defining turning point of Vesalius's life." Just when he'd achieved the pinnacle of professional achievement he threw it away, settling for a position in the imperial service which reduced him to being a military surgeon, destroying his identity as a scholar and losing his intellectual freedom.

> *Unable to cope with the reality of receiving exactly what he had to leave behind not only his academic life but also his own awaiting potential, Vesalius was overcome with madness and grief, causing him to throw his precious notes, labored drawings and treasured books into the fire. Understanding fully that his life [no] longer was his own, but someone else's. Vesalius surrendered that part of himself that he most identified with, and effectively killed it. By burning his work, Vesalius destroyed his identity as a scholar and an anatomist and assuming the*

> *role of tragic hero, was forced to reconcile with the impossible reality that he had turned away from his own destiny.*

From this rash act it is clear that young Vesalius had a keen sense of what was politically correct and it would not be surprising if he might "restrain" himself when describing his Jewish friend in the second edition. Nutton remarked that deletions may be as significant about an author as his additions, "It is not always easy to see why some passages have been left out, when others of a similar nature have been left in." Certainly in the overheated climate of the period discretion was the better part of valor; yet, as O'Malley noted, "the fact that Lazarus was mentioned at all in the later edition is fairly good-evidence, according to the practice of Vesalius, that he [Lazarus] was still alive and the two men were on amiable terms."

Of itself, that would seem remarkable since the shift in religious attitudes toward stricter orthodoxy made the outlook dire for anyone who publicly said, wrote or did anything which might be construed as heretical. But there was a perfectly reasonable alternative explanation for the deletion, for by the time that the second edition was written Lazarus, now Giovanni, no longer was Jewish! He'd converted sometime in 1549, six years after the first edition of the *Fabrica* appeared and at about the same time that Vesalius was beginning to work on a second edition. But by now Vesalius was off with the imperial court in northern Europe and may not even have known what had happened to his friend.

When Philip II and his court moved to Madrid, Vesalius moved with them, never again to return for long to Italy nor to his homeland – and now things became much worse. As described by James Ball,

> *The hand of the Church was heavy on the land; the dagger of the Inquisition was stabbing at all mental life, and its torch was a sterilizing flame sweeping all intellectual activity. The pursuit of knowledge had become a crime and to search with the scalpel was accounted sacrilege.*

There was no opportunity to perform a dissection nor even obtain a skull and jealous Spanish court physicians were hostile. It was rumored that Vesalius had mistakenly started dissecting a still living patient. Historians have refuted this story and whatever the true reason, the by now fifty year old court physician felt the need to leave Spain. As is well known, except for the details, in 1564 Vesalius sailed to the Holy Land on what was described as a "pilgrimage" – some suggested that it was penance. On the stormy return trip his ship may have been damaged and he was cast ashore on the Greek isle of Zante where he died, some historians suggest as a result of scurvy, and was buried in an unmarked grave.

WHAT KIND OF MAN WAS VESALIUS?

Historians have employed numerous adjectives to describe the anatomist's temperament: choleric, impetuous, disputatious, cocksure, extroverted, sarcastic, wrathful, schizoid, taciturn, melancholy, avaricious, having an artistic temperament. A provocative (but unsigned) essay *Vesalius the Man* argued that "except for the glorious *Fabrica* and *Epitome* nothing by Vesalius would be any loss to science."

> *There is the problem. Why was the unique genius of the man fertile only for three or four years? How came it that the greatest exponent of science of his century abandoned his career for a place at court? What sort of character can we descry through the fog of eulogy and legend and sheer hero worship? He was clearly not a man of many friends.... He had some repellant traits; in his later years he was secretive and eccentric and may even have been semi-insane. He was certainly vain and boastful, and as a writer had most of the faults of the humanists and few of their virtues. His worst feature, perhaps, came out in his ambition for he abandoned, as have many a great scientific career, for the measly reflected glamour of a life at court.*

His former mentor Sylvius had called Vesalius "a ridiculous madman" for daring to criticize the immortal Galen. Historian Stephen Joffe also referred to him as a madman suffering an identity crisis who rashly burned his works in a self-destructive act. So we have the parallel ironies of Vesalius burning his own books when he joined the Imperial court and Lazarus burning Jewish holy books when he converted to the Christian faith.

WAS THERE A JEWISH CONNECTION?

Andreas Vesalius' Christian identity was secure. Nevertheless, during Inquisition times suspicions were rife of any taint of Jewish blood. According to his own writing, Vesalius' Flemish roots, mostly from Wesel in Cleves, dated back at least to the early 15th century; three generations of his ancestors were court physicians and his father was chief apothecary for Charles V. Such *bona fides* didn't guarantee that lurking somewhere in a family's history there might have been a Jewish connection but in the case of Andreas Vesalius there is absolutely no such evidence, his sympathetic reference to his friend Lazarus notwithstanding.

Nevertheless, two of Vesalius' medical contemporaries had post-mortem surprises. In 1553 Michael Servetus (a.k.a. Villeneuve), who had been a fellow student of Vesalius in Paris, was burned at the stake in Geneva for his public stance against Calvinism and later, for good measure, was burned again in effigy by the Catholic Inquisition. More than four centuries later modern scholarship proved that Servetus was descended on his mother's side from a prominent Jewish family of Aragon. Similarly, the corpse of the famous Portuguese *converso* Garcia d'Orta (1501-1568) was exhumed twelve years after his natural death in Goa when a relative confessed under torture to continued Judaizing and implicated his cousin. An *auto da fe* was performed and d'Orta's ashes thrown into the sea.

Such narratives could have come straight out of *Candide* but unlike Voltaire's naïve Dr. Pangloss, the pragmatic Andreas Vesalius was well aware of the perilous world in which he lived and avoided mixing anatomy with theology. As for his friend Lazarus, by the time that the second edition of the *Fabrica* was written, he had opted out of his religion and, as Giovanni, would be obliged by the Inquisition to provide home care for his demented mother who hadn't. Indeed, with all this in mind, it would seem that what "distinguished" Vesalius' friend was not his medical career nor his language skill as much as his virulent public denunciation of his own Jewish roots.

2. WHO REALLY WROTE "THE PRAYER OF MAIMONIDES"?

Adapted from my book "The Jewish Doctor. A Narrative History." (1996)

Surely the most illustrious medieval Jewish physician in Arab lands was Moses Maimonides (*Rambam*) who was born in Cordova, Spain in 1135. When he was thirteen years old his family fled from a fanatical invading Islamic group (the Almohads) and wandered for more than a decade before settling in Fostat, a suburb of Cairo. At an early age he became an acclaimed interpreter of Torah and Talmud but for economic reasons he embarked on a career in medicine which culminated as a physician in the Sultan's court. He was a prolific medical writer and composed at least ten books that were written in Arabic for general consumption. His approach to treatment was always based upon common sense and personal observation and he was admired by his peers - variously described by contemporaries as "the most distinguished of his time, both in theory and in practice" and as "the eagle of physicians."

In the modern era Maimonides is best known as the presumed author of a sublime *Physicians Prayer* which William Osler described as "one of the most precious documents of our profession, worthy to be placed beside the Hippocrates oath." Indeed, sometimes the prayer is read at medical school graduation ceremonies instead of the more famous Hippocratic Oath. However, Osler had doubts about the prayer's provenance and wrote to Dr. Joseph Hertz, the chief rabbi of Great Britain, for his opinion. After due investigation, Dr. Hertz replied that the prayer was the product of an 18th century German physician Markus Herz (no relation to the rabbi) who was a friend and pupil of Immanuel Kant and Moses Mendelssohn. He worked at the Jewish Hospital in Berlin and the prayer was composed by him in the German language in 1783. An English translation first appeared in 1841 and here are a few brief excerpts from that translation:

> *May the love of my art inspire me at all times...Grant that my patients have confidence in me and my art and follow my directions and counsel...O God, Thou hast formed the body of man with infinite goodness. Thou has united in him immeasurable forces necessarily at work like so many instruments so as to preserve in its entirety this beautiful house containing his immortal soul, and these forces act with all the order and harmony imaginable..... O God, Thou has appointed me to watch over the health of Thy creatures, here am I ready for my vocation. Support me in this great task so that it may benefit mankind for without Thy help not even the least thing will succeed.*

Who was Markus Herz and why the confusion? To be mentioned in the same context as Maimonides he must have been a man of great intellect and sensitivity. The following is extracted from a biographical study by Brigitte Ibing:

> *Herz was born in 1747 in Berlin at a time when the Jewish population was living in the city illegally. His father was an impoverished Torah scribe who provided the young man with a yeshiva education. At age fifteen he moved to Koenigsberg with the intention of becoming a merchant. He had the good fortune to befriend the prosperous and highly cultivated Friedlander family and became a protege of Joachim Moses Friedlander. The youth attended Kant's lectures and began to study medicine which was the only field of higher study then open to Jews. His studies in philosophy led him to the idea that natural and humanistic sciences should be integrated and he urged that subjects like zoology and botany should be limited in favor if what today would be called psychology or psychosomatic medicine. He found it to be unsatisfactory that the universities were able to find professors who knew every bone and ligament, but not one who could teach medical psychology.* (*Koroth* 9 (1985): 113-121.)

Markus Herz strove to introduce understanding of the patient's psyche into his own medical practice in Berlin where he worked from 1774 until his death at age 56 in 1803.

He became successful and often visited up to thirty patients a day, mostly on foot, and treated regardless of social class. In addition to private practice, along with his father-in-law, he headed the Jewish Hospital and under their humane leadership the hospital developed an excellent reputation for, among other things, its cleanliness, a rare quality in those times. Although himself not religiously observant, Herz arranged for strict Jewish dietary and ceremonial laws. He tried to devise a coherent framework of applying reason in medical matters which he called "philosophical medicine." He thought of medicine as "philosophy at work," for both the individual and for society; needless to say, his ideas embroiled him in controversy among his brethren.

Dr. Herz was a leader in Berlin's Jewish Enlightenment and as an empirical scientist he was skeptical about any form of institutionalized religion. Like his friend Moses Mendelssohn, Herz believed that by introducing secular culture he thought that Judaism could be reformed and when given the opportunity to be like Germans, Jews would be accepted as such. Beginning in 1776 he and his beautiful and brilliant wife Henrietta held lectures in their home concerning science, physics, philosophy and logic. In the audience were leading intellectuals and members of the royal house, including the crown prince. The same prince became Friedrich Wilhelm II who in 1787 appointed Herz as the first Jewish professor of medicine in Prussia.

But what about the prayer that often has been attributed to Maimonides? In 1783 a *Physician's Prayer* was published anonymously in a German magazine. The full title was *Daily Prayer of a Physician From a Hebrew Manuscript of a Famous Jewish Physician in 12th century Egypt.* Of course this perfectly described who was well known in 18th century Germany, but the journal's editors provided no indication of the author's identity. Although the subject caused much controversy, most modern scholars suspect a much later author. If the work was written by Herz or someone else long after Maimonides, the reason for the deception is unclear but certain sentiments expressed in the prayer, such as "the mind of man is ever expanding," were typical of the Enlightenment spirit of optimism and improvement. After thoroughly reviewing the subject, the authoritative Dr. Fred Rosner concluded that "the physician's prayer attributed to Maimonides is a spurious work, not written by Maimonides, but composed by an 18th century writer, probably Marcus Herz. Absolute proof is, however, lacking and may never be discovered."

Some traditionalists may still maintain that Maimonides composed the *Physician's Prayer*, but whether Markus Herz wrote it or merely translated an earlier prayer from Hebrew into German, he surely was an impressive and worthy figure in his own right who strove to introduce spirituality and psychology into medical theory and practice.

3. ZOMBIE MEDICINE

Adapted from a lecture given at Saint Peters University Hospital, New Brunswick, NJ, March 10, 2015

A physician friend of mine, Dr. Philip Sarrel, introduced me to an expression that I believe he'd coined – "zombie medicine." He was aware that economist Paul Krugman sometimes uses the zombie metaphor to describe "a proposition that has been thoroughly refuted by analysis and evidence and should be dead – but won't stay dead." (NYT Oct. 14, 2013) My friend suggested that in a medical context the metaphor implies adherence to entrenched thinking despite good evidence to the contrary; flawed concepts that are difficult to eradicate – unstoppable, like a zombie plodding ahead, still stalking the land. Medical history provides many examples of clinging to incorrect doctrines For example, William Heberden's classic description of angina pectoris (1768) included only three women out of nearly one hundred cases and about a century later, William Osler wrote that angina is a rare disease which occurs "almost exclusively in men." Such authoritative statements delayed recognition of the true prevalence of this heart disorder in women until relatively recently.

Since time immemorial gullible people have fallen prey to unscrupulous charlatans and hucksters and our own time is no exception: witness such familiar fads as copper bracelets, coffee enemas and the like. Health spas still have adherents who regularly "take the waters", homeopathy has its devoted followers and cupping continues to be popular in parts of Asia – and Brooklyn. But of particular concern is when doctors themselves are deluded – not by hokum, or false claims, but by what they believe to be valid science and when respected medical authorities promote treatments, people usually listen -- credentials lend credibility.

Certainly the King of the Zombies was Galen of Pergamon (b. 130 A.D.) who taught that health or illness were a matter of balance between four fundamental "humors." If one of them got the upper hand, the proper corrective was to restore its opposite and although the concept was entirely based on speculation, it persisted for nearly two millennia. During the Middle Ages Galen was considered infallible – to criticize him was near heresy. In 1543 when Andreas Vesalius dared to question Galen's anatomic findings that were based mainly on dissections of monkeys, his former mentor Jacobus Sylvius raged that he was "a madman…whose pestilential breath poisons Europe." But Vesalius was not a lone voice against Galenic hegemony; among those before him was the rebellious Swiss alchemist Paracelsus who advocated directly observing nature rather than relying upon ancient texts, and burned Galen's books.

During the 18th century, the goal of so-called "heroic" treatment continued to be to balance opposing forces and especially to rid the ailing body of bad humors. This country's leading exponent was the versatile Benjamin Rush whose favorite regimen was to "bleed, blister, puke and purge." Few patients escaped either his lancet or his fearsome "thunderbolts" -- giant pills composed of equal parts of calomel (mercurous chloride) and jalep, both potent laxatives which presumably would expel toxic bile. Rush patented the concoction and if using his bilious pills didn't necessarily cure, at least recipients knew that they'd been treated – after all their teeth were likely to fall out from mercury toxicity. When a visiting English physician William Cobbett remarked that during a yellow fever epidemic Dr. Rush killed more people than he cured, the offended Philadelphian successfully sued for libel and Cobbett scurried home before having to pay the $8,000 fine. Indeed the true heroes of Benjamin Rush's brand of "heroic medicine" were those who survived it.

Of many medical zombies who ruled the earth during the early 19th century, perhaps the most ferocious was Francois Broussais. When he died in 1838, an obituary noted "we may safely enroll the name of Broussais among the glories of France." Yet his name is hardly remembered today. His major claim to fame was as founder of what Broussais called "physiological medicine" which emphasized the importance of function rather than pathologic anatomy. According to his theory all diseases were due to "irritability" of tissues, the "cry of suffering organs" aggravated by excessive bleeding and hyper-stimulation caused by chemical agents. There were no specific diseases, clinical signs and symptoms were merely the end-result of chronic unrecognized inflammation. In a way, "Broussaism" was a variant of Galenic theory -- if not imbalance of four humors then "irritation" as a unitary explanation for almost anything, from fever to flatulence. The way to restore physiologic balance was seductively simple: a near starvation diet, judicious use of antiphlogistics (anti-inflammatory medicines) and bleeding – not by lancet but by leech. Sometimes called "The Prince of Leeching," Broussais so captured the day that during the 1830s on average 60 million leeches were used each year – and in 1832 when France ran out of the local variety it imported forty million annelids and an international Leech Trade emerged to meet insatiable global demands. Francoise Broussais denounced all prior medical systems from the time of Hippocrates and Galen to his own day and his sarcasm directed against rivals could be brutal. He described Laennec's new stethoscope as a "useless curiosity" and as for the despised English:

> *They should stop gorging themselves with tea, alcohol and too substantial food. Their doctors should abstain from purging them at every instance…they should confine themselves to combatting the inflammation by a few capillary haemorrhages [leeches] and one would no longer see in their country such a large amount of engorgement, spleen, hypochondria, melancholy and dropsy which shorten the lives of the youngest and most robust. It is chronic enteritis, that unrecognized and badly treated disease, which depopulates England.*

During the 1820s one of his students wrote, "Monsieur Broussais is unquestionably the most remarkable medical writer of the present age. Splendid works, celebrated lectures, and a great number of proselytes, have in a few years spread far and wide his name and opinions." The great man agreed, acknowledging that his doctrine had earned "the grand astonishment and admiration of the world." He predicted that it soon would "exert an influence more marked than that exerted by vaccination" but the results were disappointing and Broussais was accused by rivals of falsifying his claims.

By 1833 when Oliver Wendell Holmes (1809-1894) arrived in Paris for two years of post-graduate study, Broussais' reputation was in eclipse, his authority eroded by younger members of the faculty who exposed the absurdities of his doctrine and the consequences of treatment by starvation and leeching. Years later Holmes recalled:

> *Broussais was in those days like an old volcano which has pretty nearly used up its fire and brimstone, but is still boiling and bubbling in its interior, and now and then sends up a spurt of lava and volley of pebbles. His theories of gastroenteritis, of irritation and inflammation as the cause of disease, and the practice which sprang from them ran over the fields of medicine for a time like flame over grass of the prairies...Broussais' theories languished and well-nigh became obsolete, and this no doubt added vehemence to his defense of his cherished dogmas.*

Although the "savage old man" Broussais was spent by the 1830s, Oliver Wendell Holmes had other notables, past and present, to criticize. With Benjamin Rush clearly in mind, he recalled that "the lancet was the magician's wand of the dark ages of medicine. The old physicians not only believed in its general efficacy as a wonder-worker in disease, but they believed that each malady could be attacked from some special part of the body – the strategic point that commanded the seat of the morbid affection." Holmes also had contemporary zombies to confront beside the burnt out likes of Rush and Broussais – indeed he was the nemesis of all zombies.

Oliver Wendell Holmes and other young Americans in Paris were captivated with the emerging French enthusiasm for "therapeutic nihilism" – it was preferable to allow nature to heal then to prescribe useless or injurious remedies; doctors should wait watchfully and supportively for the illness to run its course. As Holmes famously said, "if the whole *materia medica* as now used, could be sunk to the bottom of the sea, it would be so much the better for mankind – and all the worse for the fishes." The American students idolized their mentor Pierre Louis whose statistical analyses proved that bloodletting was ineffective, but their orthodox brethren back home sneered at this effete French passivity -- what was needed was to "break" disease." Nevertheless, by mid-19th century the skeptics prevailed and the aggressive style of treatment gave way to one of moderation. When the so-called "regulars" were forced to acknowledge that the outcomes of their approach often were no better than those of the "irregulars," many patients turned to purveyors of alternative approaches:

eclectics, herbalists, botanists, hydropaths, vegetarians, spiritualists. Then, as now, the popular justification was that at least "it can't hurt" – not very different from Galen's injunction to "do no harm."

Although the German physician Samuel Hahnemann (1755-1843) never visited the United States, his doctrine of homeopathic medicine had an enormous impact and more staying power than Broussaism. Starting in about 1796, the scholarly but outspoken Hahnemann began lambasting traditional practitioners, whom he derided as "allopaths," and designed his own medicinal substances which consisted of infinitesimal amounts of drugs diluted with alcohol and elaborately mixed and rubbed. Hocus Pocus. In 1843, the same year that Hahnemann died, Holmes scoffed that homeopathy was "a mingled mass of perverse ingenuity, of tinsel erudition, of imbecile credulity, and of artful misrepresentation." The introduction to his speech to the Boston Society for the Diffusion of Useful Knowledge titled "Homeopathy and Its Kindred Delusions" revealed the self-styled "Autocrat of the Breakfast Table" at his sarcastic best:

> *When a physician attempts to convince a person, who has fallen into the Homeopathic delusion, of the emptiness of its pretensions, he is often answered by a statement of cases in which its practitioners are thought to have effected wonderful cures...Those kind friends who suggest to a person suffering from a tedious complaint that he "Had better try Homeopathy," are apt to enforce their suggestion by adding that "at any rate it can do no harm." This may or may not be true as regards the individual. But it always does very great harm to the community to encourage ignorance, error or deception in a profession which deals with the life and health of our fellow-creatures...It may be thought that a direct attack upon the pretensions of Homeopathy is an uncalled for aggression upon an unoffending doctrine and its peaceful advocates. But a little inquiry will show that it has long assumed so hostile a position with respect to the Medical Profession, that any trouble that I, or any other member of that profession, may choose to bestow upon it may be considered merely a matter of self-defense.*

Oliver Wendell Holmes went on to rebut each of Hahnemann's "delusions" in seventy-four pages but, his words notwithstanding, by the late 19th century almost ten thousand healers practiced homeopathic medicine, 10% of all doctors nationwide. Its popularity was greatest among the country's influential and wealthy, and why not? After all, it was gentle and seemed to be based on scientific sounding principles. Moreover, homeopaths encouraged such common sense activities as eating well, exercising vigorously, fresh air and sunshine while orthodox physicians spent their time promoting bleeding and purging. To defend against incursions by economic competitors, in 1847 the "regulars" (including Holmes) formed the American Medical Association which promptly banned members from comporting with homeopaths and their ilk. However, the orthodox physicians were divided in their own house and some surgeons were happy to accept referrals from the unworthy homeopaths.

Another time Holmes spoke to the Boston Society for Medical Improvement about "The Contagiousness of Puerperal Fever" but because it was published in the obscure *New England Quarterly Journal of Medicine and Surgery* it attracted little attention. He argued that physicians' unwashed hands were responsible for transmitting puerperal fever from patient to patient which, naturally, enraged many of his colleagues. A leading obstetrician of the time Philadelphia's Charles D. Meigs scoffed that these were the "jejeune and fizzenless dreamings" of a sophomoric writer.

Four years later, another young iconoclast, Hungarian-born Ignatz Semmelweis published much the same findings concerning preventable maternal deaths. In a controlled experiment he found that having obstetricians wash their hands in a chlorinated-lime solution dropped maternal mortality from 10% to below 1%. He, too, was derided by the medical establishment and, for him personally, the result was tragic. Semmelweis lost his hospital position, was forced to move from Vienna to Budapest and when he wrote angry letters accusing European obstetricians of being irresponsible murderers, he was said to be insane (even his wife agreed.) No doubt he was unbalanced to a degree and in 1865 the forty-seven year old physician was forcibly committed to an asylum. He died there two weeks later, possibly as a result of injuries sustained when beaten by guards, and it wasn't for nearly another three decades as a result of Pasteur's work that Ignatz Semmelweis's findings gained acceptance. In our time, reference sometimes is made to a so-called "Semmelweis Reflex" or "Semmelweiss Effect" which refers to a tendency to automatically reject new knowledge that contradicts established beliefs – in effect, "zombie medicine."

Given the choice of accepting empirical evidence or clinging to misguided or mindless beliefs, many people, if not most, would choose the latter. A case in point was "autointoxication," an ancient theory based on the belief that putrifying waste products located in the intestines can poison the body and are a major contributor to most diseases. The concept had a revival during the 19th century when colonic irrigation achieved what has been described as "a triumph of ignorance over science." Among those who encouraged an aggressive approach to promote health and "cleanse the body of filth" was a dour Presbyterian minister in Bound Brook, New Jersey, Sylvester Graham (1794-1851) who had a stern message: "If it feels good, don't do it." Graham advocated hard mattresses, open bedroom windows, vigorous exercise – and chastity – but equally important was a high fiber vegetarian diet. He developed a biscuit made from molasses and whole wheat flour that had no additives that's still with us today: the Graham cracker! When introduced in 1829 he claimed that regular use would cure indigestion, poor circulation, insanity --and also would reduce lust.

That message must have appealed to Dr. John Harvey Kellogg (1852-1943) another food faddist who also was engaged in "warfare with passion." Adopting some of Graham's natural ways of promoting health, he opened a "University of Health" in Battle Creek Michigan that was staffed by 800 to 1,000 and treated a wealthy and celebrity clientele. Patients at his sanitarium were kept busy sunbathing, doing breathing exercises, eating Corn Flakes and, most important, having frequent enemas because he believed that 90% of illness originated there. A special machine could instill 15 gallons within a few seconds. This was followed by purifying yogurt – half by mouth, half per rectum – and the result was a "squeaky clean" colon.

The yogurt idea was adopted from the Russian immunologist Elie Metchnikoff (1845-1916), director of the Pasteur Institute and Nobel Laureate in 1908. He favored the magical properties of a drink popular among Bulgarian peasants that was made from fermented yogurt (*kefir*) that contained lactic acid. When ingested regularly it would normalize gastrointestinal flora (like today's probiotics), improve digestion, enhance the immune system and slow the aging process. But Metchnikoff and Kellogg differed over just what to eat. The Russian feared that raw food contained dangerous microbes and was an unreconstructed flesh-eater. In describing "Metchnikoff's Mistake" Kellogg wrote that he "eats a pound of meat and lets it rot in his colon and then drinks a pint of sour milk to disinfect it. I am not such a fool. I don't eat meat." Metchnikoff drank sour milk every day of his life until his death in 1916 at the age of 71; Graham groused that this was premature, that he would have lived longer if he wasn't a carnivore.

The death blow to Galen's old zombie should have occurred with publication of Rudolph Virchow's *Cellular Pathology* (1858) and the advent of Pasteur's germ theory, but it didn't entirely happen. Broussais' discredited theory reemerged transformed -- the culprit shifting from irritation/inflammation to infection. In 1900, the British surgeon William Hunter identified "oral sepsis" as a cause of a multitude of diseases. Soon Frank Billings in Chicago was claiming that tonsillectomies and dental extractions cured "focal infection" which otherwise might effect distant organs. Charles Mayo and other luminaries supported the theory and by 1930 excision of focal infections was considered a rational form of therapy thought to resolve many cases of chronic disease.

Starting about 1908 the acclaimed English surgeon Sir W. Arbuthnot Lane (1856-1943) took a novel approach to "colonic inertia" by performing colectomies. Arguing that modern society was ruining health, he promoted sunlight, physical exercise and a high fiber diet which could prevent cancer. By the 1920s Lane abandoned total colectomies in favor of a modified procedure: lysis of what he described as congenital bands of adhesions in the bowel wall which contributed to constipation, stasis and "flooding the circulation with filthy material." Dr. Lane developed a loyal following and a profitable society practice, but fell into disfavor with many of his medical colleagues. He abandoned practice to market a redesigned toilet to create a more "natural" position for the prolonged colonic ablutions that were necessary two or three times every day. Today, "Lane's Disease" is still in vogue, listed as a cause of chronic constipation with colectomy prescribed to treat refractory cases.

Perhaps the most zealous American proponent of Lane's "surgical bacteriology" was Dr. Henry Cotton (1876-1933), medical director of the Trenton State Hospital, who identified focal infection as the main cause of schizophrenia, manic depression and masturbation. The challenge was to locate the offending pocket of pus and the most convenient starting point was the mouth. Beginning in 1916 Dr. Cotton began removing his mentally disturbed patients' teeth and tonsils even if there were no abnormal signs and, if that didn't do the job, he probed deeper and removed internal organs: gall bladders, spleens, reproductive organs. If abdominal X-rays revealed retention of fecal matter or if the patient suffered from constipation, he would remove their entire colon. In one twelve month period there were 6.472 dental extractions performed at Trenton State Hospital, 542 tonsillectomies and 79 colectomies. He claimed up to 85% cure rate and justified one third mortality of colectomized patients because this radical procedure was done only as "a last resort" for end-stage patients. Cotton believed his own theory enough that he extracted both of his sons' teeth – each of them later committed suicide.

Some called Henry Cotton "the new Lister." The president of the New Jersey Medical Society proclaimed, "Dr. Cotton has built a foundation for the benefit of the health of the people of which every succeeding generation will reap the benefits and generations to come will rise up and call him blessed." The president of the AMA proclaimed Trenton State to be "one of the country's great institutions…a monument to the most advanced civilization of her people." A reporter for the New York Times enthused that Cotton's brilliant work was "the most searching, aggressive and profound scientific investigation that has as yet been made in the whole field of mental and nervous disorders." But his results seemed to good to be true and, finally, an independent investigator who reviewed the records of 645 major operative cases done between 1918 and 1932 found disturbing results: mortality of 44.7% (138/309) for those receiving colectomies; 13.7% of 336 who were given Lane's "pericolonic membranotomies" and there were many fewer "cures" than Dr. Cotton had reported. But long after his theory was discredited, surgical attacks on presumably infected teeth and tonsils continued unabated. Millions of tonsils were sacrificed prophylactically in order to eliminate focal infection and even today some advocates of "biological dentistry" recommend tooth extraction and oral surgery to remove foci of infection which presumably might cause systemic disease. Once again, it was difficult to slay the zombie.

During the late 19th and early 20th centuries Europe was a hotbed of zombies. In 1889 the distinguished French physician Charles Brown-Sequard read a paper at a scientific meeting in Paris which shocked the audience. He described how over a period of two weeks he'd injected himself with a solution of ground testicles of dogs and guinea pigs and noted a marked increase both in strength and stamina, improved mental energy and regular bowel movements: "All has changed and I have regained the full force that I possessed." These salubrious effects persisted for about a month after the last injection and then wore off. To his credit, Brown-Sequard made his data available for all to review and refused to endorse any products capitalizing on his discovery. But that didn't deter others. Russian-born Serge Voronoff popularized grafting monkey testicles into human scrotums with astonishing rejuvenative results. When the Viennese physiologist Eugen Steinach theorized that ligation of the vas deferens would cause testicular secretions to "back up" resulting in improved vigor, potency, hair growth and eyesight, people clamored to be "steinached." Irish poet William Butler Yeats lauded his "second puberty" but Sigmund Freud was less enthusiastic with his own response. "Glandular fever" gradually abated but not before an American huckster William "Doc" Brinkley (see chapter 14) became fabulously wealthy grafting goat testes into failing males – he promised to make "every man the ram that am with every lamb." Although the monkey business eventually fell out of favor, current enthusiasm for testosterone injections is evidence that this zombie still has life.

All medical zombies are not dead yet! Some are hidden in plain sight – stubborn to the end. Ancient methods of cupping and acupuncture have great staying power and still are widely used. The Food and Drug Administration permits sale of leeches for use in microsurgery to relieve venous congestion and has supported research to explore its value in different diseases. Vitamin and supplements sales exceed $11 billion a year while homeopathy's proponents claim over 200 million followers worldwide. Infected gums and teeth as the cause of systemic disease still has serious supporters and the beneficial use of cleansing enemas persists in the public mind. More than a century after Elie Metchnikoff's observations about the efficacy of yogurt, we are witnessing a boom in the use of probiotics ("good germs") being marketed to improve health. Indeed, there's current enthusiasm for fecal transplants to treat ileitis and colitis.

Social historians like to study how changing notions of illness reflect prevailing cultural conditions – how and why what's considered "wrong" now once seemed "right." More important is how in the future we will respond when what's now considered "right" proves to be "wrong." To this day many people, including physicians, are reluctant to change their beliefs after previously accepted ideas have been proven to be incorrect. If medical history teaches nothing else, it should be that zombies exist in all times and a continuing challenge is to discover where they are hidden. Where are our zombies?

4. PLAGUES AND POX

Adapted from a lecture given at LIU's Adult Learning Collaborative, Orangeburg, NY, September 18, 2014.

Few of us usually give much thought to infectious diseases. At birth we enter a sterile environment and within seconds of opening our eyes antibiotics are dropped in. We drink pure water and pasteurized milk, bathe or shower every day and are urged to wash our hands frequently. Doctors prescribe antibiotics – perhaps too often – and most of us dutifully renew our Flu shots every year. Public Health usually is left to the professionals, but this summer (2014) came news about Ebola virus and part of that story has been that the professionals weren't up to the task. We've heard how some local behavior has been heroic and some horrendous but, as we'll soon see, in certain respects human behavior hasn't changed all that much from the past. Ebola aside, most years, except on cruise ships or during flu season, we don't worry about epidemics and the question is have we grown too complacent? Most senior citizens remember summer polio scares but can you imagine what life must have been like long before anyone knew about germ theory – no less antisepsis and antibiotics?

Throughout most of human history people lived in fear of disease. Every decision had to be made under the shadow of death: a farm family needed many children lest they became short-handed; to appoint a godparent was more than an honorific -- it was a practical kind of insurance – just in case. Medical science depended on received wisdom rather than based on clinical observation or experimentation. Some people believed that epidemics were divine punishment. Others thought they were due to some celestial event -- a passing comet, an earthquake. Perhaps it was a curse by witches or gypsies or Jews. Poisoned wells? The Evil Eye? Satan? And when things got really serious, human reactions included panic, prayer, penance, hedonism, stoicism, scapegoating, animal or human sacrifice.

In his classic book *Rats, Lice and History* (1934) Hans Zinsser made the case that plagues always have and will continue to reinvent themselves while science scrambles to keep up. He focused on epidemic typhus but to Zinsser, infectious disease in general wasn't an abstraction – it was ever present and effected human history in one way or another. He wrote in an engaging style – consider this:

> *Infectious disease is one of the few genuine adventures left in the world. The dragons are all dead, and the lance grows rusty in the chimney corner.... Our own continent is a stage route of gas stations and the Indians own oil wells. Africa is a playground for animal photographers or museum administrators and their wives who go there partly to have their pictures taken with one foot on a dead lion.*

Hans Zinsser went on to say that Infectious disease is one of the "great tragedies of living things – the struggle for existence between different forms of life":

> *The only genuine sporting activity left is our war against these ferocious little fellow creatures, which lurk in the dark corners and stalk us in the bodies of rats, mice and all kinds of domestic animals; which fly and crawl with the insects, and waylay us in our food and drink -- and even in our love.*

When Pizzaro in Peru and Cortez in Mexico defeated the Aztecs and Incas during the early 16th century, it was less with their horses and guns than with their germs. Small pox wiped out millions of natives, whole villages were depopulated and the survivors meekly submitted to the superior white man's god. In North America the conquistadors infected natives not only with small pox but with typhus, measles, scarlet fever, diphtheria and other mundane European bugs – frequently 90% of the population were wiped out from this form of germ warfare. But the natives returned the favor and the conquerors brought back syphilis to the Old World – a reverse form of "Montezuma's revenge" - which quickly ravaged Europe.

Until the early 20th century there was a perception, both among the general population and among physicians themselves, that although they could comfort, doctors really couldn't cure serious illness. It wasn't until the 1870s and 80s that within a single decade the causes of leprosy, anthrax, gonorrhea, TB, rabies and malaria all were found to be caused by microorganisms most of which, after proper staining, could be seen with a simple microscope. Pasteur wrote, "It is in the power of man to rid humanity of every parasitic disease." But physicians were slow to accept these findings and it took nearly another century before antibiotics finally wiped out most of the bad bugs and vaccines built immunity against others as well as certain viruses. Now let's consider some of the most important epidemic diseases.

The term "plague was used from the 14 and 15th centuries to mean a devastating affliction or calamity. The name was derived from the Latin *plaga* – meaning a sudden blow or wound. The Biblical Ten Plagues were calamities more than infections (with the possible exception of boils) and in Hebrew the word for plagues was *makot* -- again, literally meaning a "blow." It was written in *1 Chronicles* that as a punishment for King David ordering, of all things, a census [?], God caused a severe plague which destroyed 70,000 people in one day. It's not clear what was so bad about conducting a census but the Old Testament did understand the concept of contagion – for example, lepers were kept outside the main camp lest they infect others.

The first pandemic that we know much about broke out in North Africa in 430 BC and then spread by ship to Athens. Without warning, healthy people developed fever, headache, chest and stomach symptoms and died very quickly (most likely it was due to typhus.) Athenian life was profoundly effected; people were demoralized and the army was paralyzed. In his history of the Peloponnesian Wars, Thucydides described how corpses were left unburied, religious ceremonies abandoned and lawlessness prevailed.

> *Men now cooly ventured on what they had formerly done in a corner, and did just as they pleased...They resolved to spend quickly and enjoy themselves... Perseverance in what men called honour was popular with none... It was settled that present enjoyment and all that contributed to it was both honorable and useful. Fear of gods or*

> *law of men, there was none to restrain them... It was only reasonable to enjoy life a little"*

Or as Isaiah said, "Live today for tomorrow we may die." The same pattern of behavior occurred in most subsequent plagues. About a millennium after the so-called Plague of Athens, the Roman Empire headed by Emperor Justinian was based in Constantinople (Byzantium). In 541 AD the capital was devastated by what a Greek historian described as "a pestilence by which the whole human race came near to being annihilated." Well not quite, however some 40% of the population died; Emperor Justinian himself was stricken but recovered – and many historians attributed the fall of the Roman Empire to this epidemic of plague.

Fast forward about another eight centuries to the 1340s when plague returned to Europe and wiped out between 30 and 70% of the population – some 25 million people! It was popularly known as the Black Death because of horrible necrotic skin lesions, and starting in 1601, it was called Bubonic Plague because of the characteristic "buboes" which were swollen lymph nodes in the neck, armpits, groin or internally, some the size of grapefruits. Now we know that the culprits were rats which served as hosts for fleas which, in turn, carried a bacterium with a lethal punch (endotoxin.) But nobody knew that for another 500 years.

The Black Death began in Asia, travelled westward and over about five years spread all over Europe and the Middle East. Some scholars believe it was carried by invading Mongol horsemen but back then most people thought that it was God's doing – people's attention was directed upward rather than down at their feet. Starting in Venice as early as 1377, incoming ships were quarantined for forty days at a Lazaretto on an off shore island before they could unload; it was a semi-effective means of controlling transmission from what they knew not. Unlike other familiar diseases, plague killed quicker. Europe's population was drastically reduced and it took a century or more to recover. Of course this effected the economy because there were fewer workers and the good news for survivors was that job opportunities and salaries increased. There was redistribution of wealth and for the first time governments began establishing policies which emphasized public good, even if they impinged on individual rights.

Although doctors had no answers they pretended they did and profited. Gravediggers also prospered. To be sure there were acts of charity but also instances of cruelty and lawlessness. Thousands of the pious marched in penitential parades from city to city; some flagellated themselves; others burned Jews – sometimes prophylactically when plague was nearby – and at times there were mass dancing manias. Some people said that extreme rest was therapeutic – just smell flowers and listen to soothing music - but those who could fled, abandoning homes and possessions. The dictum was "flee early, flee far, return late." Cities built walls and locked the gates; vigilantes armed with pitchforks patrolled the roads to keep out strangers and those caught escaping from quarantined cities sometimes were shot or hung. Everyone avoided the sick – often ill servants or even family members were forced out, laws were abandoned and sexual morality loosened.

Cities were full of corpses, bodies placed at the curb to be carted away. When churches ran out of graves they dug huge trenches and corpses were dumped in without ceremony, squashed down and covered with lime. If graves were too shallow, dogs would dig them up and gnaw on the bodies and in the worst of times corpses were piled up along the seashore to wash away. As one person recalled, "There were none who wept for any death, for everyone expected to die." During the Middle Ages, people wore charms and amulets and masks with strange bird-like beaks that were stuffed with aromatics – eerily similar looking to the biohazard gear that Ebola workers currently wear.

Every plague had its chronicler. In the time of Justinian it was Thucydides but during the Black Death in 14th century Florence it was Boccaccio. In his famous work the *Decameron* ten people fearing for their lives and camped out in church decided to pass the time by each telling one story every day for 10 days – the result was 100 tales, Decameron. Later writers whom I'll describe included the likes of Daniel DeFoe and Albert Camus, but the most famous description was contained in the beloved nursery rhyme *Ring Around the Rosie:*

Ring around the Rosie,
A pocketful of posies,
Ashes, Ashes,
We all fall down.

Presumably the ring around the rosie referred to the plague's typical red rash; pockets full of posies to the practice of carrying sweet-smelling flowers in pockets both to keep away the disease and the stench; ashes were the results of cremation and "we all fall down" needs no explanation.

The most detailed account of The Great London Plague of 1665 was a journal written by Daniel DeFoe, the author of *Robinson Crusoe.* It was supposed to have been a daily journal of his own experiences, but at the time of the Great Plague DeFoe was only a small child. In fact, he wrote his so-called memoir some fifty years later knowing that it would be a guaranteed best-seller at a time when Londoners feared that still another epidemic was coming their way. He described a mass exodus of some 200,000 wealthy people out of the city which included the medical elite -- but the departing Royal College of Physicians was kind enough to leave for those remaining behind a pamphlet called "Certain Necessary Directions for the Prevention and Cure of the Plague" – and, presumably, good luck! Among their suggestions was for shut-ins to think pleasant thoughts of gold and silver rather than to brood about death. Because tobacco was thought to be protective schoolboys were forced to smoke and those who disobeyed were flogged.

During the London Plague, for the first time statistics ("Bills of Mortality") were kept about the numbers who'd died each week and, in time, these tallies evolved to our modern death certificates. Defoe described how church bells tolled incessantly, how the stench was overwhelming, how fires burned everywhere to clear the air. Madmen roamed the streets predicting doom. There were campaigns to exterminate all cats and dogs but this was counterproductive because cats and dogs killed rats which carried the fleas so the rats were ignored -- anyway there were just too many of them. Along with their families, sick people were locked in their houses which were marked by a red-cross; windows and keyholes plugged to keep the evil miasma (bad air) from escaping. Municipalities and churches provided medical supplies and food which were passed through a window by special couriers. Many people objected to being taxed to pay for those who were locked in the pest houses -- after all, it was their problem - and as Samuel Pepys wrote in his diary, "the plague makes us cruel as dogs to one another."

The last great pandemics of plague in Europe came in Marseilles in 1720 and in Moscow in 1771. In 1894 there was a pandemic limited to China -- whereas The Black Death killed about 25 million people over five years, about one third of Europe's population, the Chinese pandemic "only" killed about 13 million out of a much larger population. In 1924 there was a mild rat-related outbreak in Los Angeles and even today there are occasional reports of sporadic cases carried by infected bats in desert areas in the American West. In recent years it's been reemerging in Asia and Africa where several thousand new cases are reported to WHO every year; however, the modern strain of the bacterium is less virulent and less infectious than in the past.

In 1894 the organism which caused bubonic plague was discovered, almost simultaneously but separately, by two scientists both working in Hong Kong. One (Shiba Kitasato) was a Japanese student of Koch while the other was a Swiss student of Pasteur. In time the germ would be named after the latter, Dr. Alexander Yersin, as *Yersinia pestis* (it used to be called *Pasteurella pestis*) who discovered that although it was carried by rats it was transmitted by fleas. In recent years, DNA testing of the teeth of skeletons in mass graves from the time of the London plague confimed that *Yersinia* was the cause. There were two major bacterial variants – the most common form was bubonic plague, the less common but more lethal form (100% mortality) called pneumonic plague was the only type that could be transmitted directly from human to human via droplets of sputum; because people died so quickly, they didn't have time to develop buboes. The bubonic form required a bite from the insect vector and let's not forget that mosquitoes and other insects also transmit malaria, yellow fever, dengue, West Nile Fever, Lyme Disease, Zika and many other diseases. DDT wasn't discovered until World War II and soon was being widely used in agriculture but many insects developed resistance and in 1962 Rachel Carson's book *Silent Spring* emphasized the potential harm on the environment of indiscriminate spraying.

Long before anyone knew about the tubercle bacillus tuberculosis often was called "The White Plague." It wasn't transmitted by fleas but human to human through droplets spread by coughing or sneezing; before milk was pasteurized there also was a form called bovine tuberculosis. For centuries the disease was known as consumption or phthisis until in 1882 Robert Koch discovered the tubercle bacillus which led to the official name *mycobacterium tuberculosis*. There are other kinds of mycobacterial diseases, e.g. leprosy, but although even now roughly one third of the world population are infected; fortunately only about one tenth of them develop clinical disease.

The name White Plague referred to the fact that patients characteristically appeared pale while the term consumption was used because they literally were wasted by the disease. Usually it was a chronic disorder which seemed to attack just one person at a time. The symptoms could be subtle or entirely absent -- perhaps only a pallid complexion or flushed face, night sweats, a persistent cough, specks of blood on the pillowcase and it could last for years, even decades. Conventional wisdom was that there was a hereditary predisposition that was provoked by such things as bad air, early marriage, strong liquor, tight lacing, too much or too little exercise, lack of sleep, ill-fated love, self-abuse, winter winds, living in cellars, vampires. A recent article in the NYTimes cited DNA evidence suggesting that TB originated in Africa less than 6,000 years ago and was carried across the Atlantic to South America by infected seals where it crossed over into humans. Seals! Who knew?

Between the 13th and 18th centuries, it was believed that scrofula, the form of TB which involved swollen lymph nodes, especially in the neck, could be cured by the king's "Royal Touch" when such standard treatments as the blood of a weasel or dove's dung had failed. French kings were enthusiastic touchers but during the 17th century Charles II of England was the champion – said to have touched more than 90,000 sufferers during his long reign. Unfortunately, they didn't keep records of the outcomes back then and no one knew of double-blind studies.

When Frederic Chopin was diagnosed with the disease in 1838 he was sent to Majorca for the mild climate. The French didn't believe that TB was contagious but the locals thought differently and when they discovered that the musician was consumptive, wanted nothing to do with him. Chopin tried to hire a carriage to Palma where he could board a ship home but no one would carry him so he had to travel by wheel barrow. As his companion George Sand wrote, "We boarded the only steamship that comes to the island and which is used to transfer pigs to Barcelona. There was no other way to move out of this wretched country. At the time of leaving the inn in Barcelona, the innkeeper wanted us to pay for Chopin's bed under the pretext that it was infected and that the police had ordered burning it." This account differed considerably from the conventional narrative of Chopin's life but, even if inaccurate, differences of opinion about cause and susceptibility persisted. Even when Koch's animal experiments confirmed that the disease was contagious, he believed that what he called "the seed" wouldn't cause disease unless the "soil" was receptive – in other words, certain people were predisposed - and perhaps they are.

Novels and operas frequently were filled with gaunt, coughing, slowly dying consumptives: all the patients in Thomas Mann's *Magic Mountain,* Little Eva in *Uncle Tom's Cabin,* perhaps Jane Eyre. TB wasn't perceived as repulsive or immoral; somehow it seemed ennobling, its victims long suffering such as Violetta in *La Traviata* and Mimi in *La Boheme.* Some believed that consumption heightened the senses and spurred creativity. Among the literati thought to have TB were Jane Austen, Robert Louis Stevenson, D.H. Lawrence, Edgar Allen Poe, Emily Dickinson, Kafka, Keats, Shelley, Browning, Thoreau, Whittier, Chekhov, Moliere, Balzac - and those were just the writers.

Lacking any effective treatment, during the 1830s consumptives went to sea as sailors or whalers or voyagers. During the 1860s they went west to farm, or pan for gold, or to live a strenuous outdoor life. During the 1870s the emphasis shifted, at least for those with advanced disease. The sanatorium movement which began in Europe was based on the principle that TB could be treated by rest, fresh air and plenty of sunshine. Resorts flourished in the mountains of Switzerland and the pine forests of Finland where life was tightly regulated by the medical staff and the chief administrator was called the Superintendent -- an apt term because he commanded every aspect of life within his domain. Patients were virtual prisoners; they were there to follow orders. Nevertheless there was an illicit underground culture of death -- breaking rules, covert sexual alliances as described in *The Magic Mountain.* Dr. Edward Trudeau claimed to have cured his own tuberculosis by living outdoors and in 1894 opened his own sanatorium in Saranac Lake. Wealthy patients flocked there from all over, lived in so-called "cure cottages" and sat outside in specially designed Adirondack chairs for hours every day and in all seasons.

In this country during the 19th and early 20th centuries, TB was responsible for about one in five deaths - rich and poor, city or farm, young and old. Nearly half died, more than 100,000 every year – not all at once but one at a time -- and it remained the leading cause of death until early in the 20th century. When TB finally was proven to be contagious the government became actively involved in prevention – there were mandatory chest X-rays, child-labor laws, pasteurization of milk. Moreover, it was necessary for all people, not only patients, to take responsibility for their general behavior – for example: not spitting in public places and being frugal and disciplined. In truth the slow decline of TB probably owed more to public health measures, housing reform and slum clearance than to medical interventions at least until 1945 with the discovery and availability of streptomycin and other effective antibiotics.

In 1906 New Jersey passed legislation which permitted counties to establish their own isolation hospitals and sanatoria and for many years I worked at one of them -- Bergen Pines County Hospital in Paramus. During the 1920s and 30s about 80% of the patients treated there had TB and stayed an average of about 200 days. Although chest specialists advised three or four years for best results, few patients could tolerate the program and many signed out before they were considered "cured." The healing properties of sunlight had been proclaimed for thousands of years but with the advent of electricity, seemingly, nature could be improved upon by using high power ultraviolet lamps. At Bergen Pines dozens of patients lay on parallel litters, their bare bodies exposed to the bright light while wearing goggles to protect their eyes. These so-called "sun-starved" children came from inner cities and had positive skin tests but no symptoms yet. They were admitted to a special unit called the "Preventorium" where every day they received "heliotherapy" lying under sun lamps in order to boost their resistance. (Afterward they no longer looked pale but I wonder how many of them later developed skin cancer?) Nowadays the sanatoria either have been closed or converted for other purposes but there still are about 15,000 new cases of TB in this country each year and although it's treatable, resistant strains have emerged which effect immune deficient patients, especially those with AIDS, and epidemics continue in third world countries, such as Nepal and rural Russia, where TB still kills about two million people a year.

Now let's shift our attention from black and white plagues to what the English sometimes called the red plague or more commonly "the Pox." The word pox refers to the characteristic pustular rash which often left disfiguring scars – George Washington's face was said to be pockmarked, although you wouldn't know it from looking at Gilbert Stuart's flattering portraits, and so was Joseph Stalin's face. Few know that Abraham Lincoln developed a mild case of small pox, probably from his son, and was quarantined for three weeks just after delivering the Gettysburg Address. The designation SMALL Pox was first used in the 15th century to distinguish it from the equally worrisome GREAT Pox – syphilis – about which I'll speak next. A more familiar term for the disease during the 18th century was "variola" which was derived from a Latin word meaning "spotted" or "pimple." In fact the rash looked much like chicken pox except for its distribution.

But the story of immunization goes much further back. Inhalation or injection into the skin of fresh small pox material seems to have been practiced in China and India as early as the 10th century. It was common knowledge that survivors of small pox didn't have recurrences and inoculation of pus from a sick person could prevent a healthy person from contracting a serious case. The procedure known as "variolation" was introduced into the Western world because of a remarkable English woman, Lady Mary Wortley Montagu. Brilliant and beautiful, she had almost died at age 26 from a severe case of smallpox which left her badly disfigured. In 1717 her husband, who was hardly her match in cleverness, was appointed England's ambassador to Turkey and as soon as they arrived in Istanbul, Lady Montagu learned the language and became a fixture in court society. She was surprised to learn that the locals had no fear of small pox for there was an ancient custom of injecting children with pus from people with mild disease and, although they developed symptoms, none died or were scarred. So Lady Montagu had her three year old son inoculated and when she returned to England in 1718, she did the same for her daughter - and soon her influential friends at court followed suit.

Three years later, in 1721, an epidemic broke out in Boston when a ship from the West Indies landed carrying several crew members with small pox and within a few months about half of the city's 12,000 citizens became ill. The slave of Rev. Cotton Mather, the famous burner of witches, told his master about a method of inoculation used by African natives. Mather sent a letter to Boston's medical society – all twelve of them -- but they denied that anything could be learned from heathens. However there was one willing doctor Zabdiel Boylston who tried the method on his own family. There nearly was a riot and a grenade was thrown through Cotton Mather's window but before long many people voluntarily lined up to be variolated. They all developed mild symptoms but usually recovered and within a few weeks Boston was described as "one large hospital." Boylston was accused of being an illiterate fool, a murderer and worse but he kept careful records and reported that only 6 of 242 of his patients died, about 2%, compared to 14% mortality for those untreated.

Some fifty years later during the Revolutionary War there was another outbreak in Boston and those infected were sent to pest houses. If they refused, their yards were fenced in and red warning flags hung outside.

Again there was a rush to inoculate and Abigail Adams wrote to her husband in Philadelphia that "all the little folks are very sick and puke every morning but after that they are comfortable." General Washington feared that the epidemic might be deadlier than British swords and risked having his soldiers variolated even though they'd be temporarily out of action. Unaware, the British didn't take advantage. During the years of the Revolution about 130,000 people (including native Americans) died of small pox compared to about 25,000 due to military casualties – five times more from the pox than from the war - and soon variolation became wide spread. But before long use of live smallpox pus was replaced by another method. In 1796 Dr. Edward Jenner found a young dairymaid who'd caught cowpox from a cow called Blossom and inoculated material from fresh lesions on her hands into the eight year old son of his gardener. Although the boy developed mild fever and rash, about two months later when reinoculated with pus from a fresh smallpox lesion, no disease ensued. He was immune and the rest is history.

Skipping ahead about a century, in 1900 smallpox broke out in New York's tenements where there were more than a thousand cases and over 400 deaths. Health Commissioner Ernst Lederle was sent to Europe to learn new methods of prevention and treatment and when he returned set up an emergency force of 200 vaccinators who, accompanied by policemen, vaccinated more than 800,000 people within six months. The last reported naturally occurring case of smallpox in this country was in 1949, and the last in the world was in Somalia in 1977. After the disease was eradicated here, routine vaccination was stopped in 1972, but enough vaccine was stockpiled to cover everyone in case of a future emergency.

Although there are skeptics, there's a plausible theory that syphilis, once called "The Great Pox", was introduced into Europe by members of Columbus's crew who contracted it from natives on Haiti. The Admiral himself may have been a victim and some think that he died of it. When they returned home in 1493, with "more sickness than gold," some sailors became mercenaries in the French army of Charles VII when they invaded Naples. The Italians surrendered without a fight but got more than they bargained for. After their surrender, there was general carousing and then the French army dispersed to spread their spirochetes throughout Europe. Very quickly there was a devastating outbreak of the Great Pox. There was paranoia and xenophobia about who was to blame. Naturally the Italians called it French Disease while the French called it Neapolitan Disease and as the calamity spread, the Spanish blamed the Dutch, the Russians blamed the Poles, Tahitians the British, Japanese the Chinese, the Vatican blamed Jews and the Turks called it "The Christian Disease." Syphilis was the name of a shepherd who was the hero of a popular poem written in 1530 by the Italian physician Fracastoro: Syphilis was smitten with the disease after he had defied the Gods. Doctors used to refer to syphilis as *Lues* -- derived from the Latin word for plague and the spirochete that we now know to be its cause is called *Treponema pallidum.*

The symptoms were dramatic: rash, ulcerations, deformities, excruciating pain, boils and buboes, even death. During the 15th and 16th centuries the symptoms of syphilis were far worse then what later centuries experienced. One theory is that a relatively benign bacteria which caused a non-venereal disease called yaws mutated to a highly virulent form which Columbus's men brought home. Probable sufferers among the musical, artistic and literary worlds included the likes of Schubert, Schuman, Donizetti, Maupassant, Flaubert, Van Gogh, Gauguin, Goya, Wilde, Heine, Beethoven, Joyce, Nietzsche. Bad guys too: Hitler, Mussolini, Lenin, Ivan the Terrible, Al Capone. Doctors often called syphilis "The Great Imitator" because it could simulate almost anything and because the worst effects of tertiary syphilis might not appear for twenty or thirty years, some called it "the hidden plague." Of course its victims were subject to other sexually transmitted diseases as well. For example, in his famous diary James Boswell proudly described having seventeen instances of "the clap" (gonorrhea) and it seems likely that such a sociable fellow might also have contracted syphilis in someone's bed and not known about it.

It's unclear why the virulence of certain germs change over time. Syphilis and leprosy seemed to lose steam long before there were effective treatments available while, on the other hand, plague could go underground for long periods and then burst forth, seemingly for no accountable reason. The first treatments for syphilis employed mercury which wasn't particularly effective, but at least you knew you'd been treated because your teeth and hair would fall out. Then in 1905 Paul Ehrlich discovered what he called Salversan or "606" or "the magic bullet" (arsphenamine.) It was less toxic than mercury and was about all there was available until penicillin came along during World War II which changed everything.

If plague dominated the 14th through 17th centuries and small pox and yellow fever the 18th, the bacterial superstar of the 19th century was cholera – some called it "The Blue Terror" because of terminal cyanosis.

Although TB peaked about the same time and killed more people it was a chronic disease while cholera could lay out a healthy person within hours. The word cholera is derived from the Greek word for bile. It was spread by swallowing fecal matter on unwashed hands, uncooked fruits or vegetables or contaminated raw fish. Its onset was spectacular – vomiting, diarrhea, dehydration and death – people who were well in the morning often were gone before night. It couldn't be romanticized like with the lingering debility of tuberculosis, but sometimes cholera was used as a literary backdrop such as in Thomas Mann's novella *Death in Venice.* At the end of Garcia Marquez's *Love in the Time of Cholera*" (1985) when the long separated lovers are reunited late in life, they cruise down the river as the only passengers on a ship supposedly infected with cholera – they'd bribed the captain to fly the yellow flag of cholera so no one else would come on board to disturb them. They couldn't land at any port and as both the book and the movie end they sail on together – infected with love.

Before the 19th century there'd never been a large epidemic of cholera outside of the Far East but beginning in India in 1817, it spread westward. English doctors were aware that patients became severely dehydrated and in 1833, for the first time in history, they began injecting large volumes of saline solution directly into veins – sometimes with dramatic but only temporary results. The English public distrusted doctors who they believed were killing patients in order to study their bodies and there were "cholera riots" in several English cities. There also were riots against government restrictions in Russia and Germany where quarantine methods did no good because it wasn't transmitted from person to person like with pulmonary plague or small pox. Cholera appeared cyclically during the 1830s and 40s (see next chapter) and then again in 1866, each new outbreak less severe than before until it finally disappeared for good – except, of course, in the Third World.

The most dramatic medical breakthrough came in 1854 when there was a ferocious epidemic of cholera in the SoHo section of London. Within the first three days 127 people died and within two weeks fatalities reached 500 – all within a few blocks. A neighborhood doctor by the name of John Snow didn't accept conventional wisdom that cholera was related to bad air, called miasma. He suspected that it was due to bad water and, like a medical Sherlock Holmes, John Snow questioned all the locals and carefully mapped where each victim lived or worked. Every case could be traced to a single pump - what became famous as "The Broad Street

Pump" - which provided drinking water for the whole neighborhood and was located just three feet from an overflowing cesspool. Because Dr. Snow was an unknown who hadn't attended the best schools, medical authorities were slow to accept his idea but it couldn't be denied that the epidemic was snuffed out as soon as the pump's handle was removed.

John Snow's investigations helped lead to improved water supplies and today he's credited as being "the father of epidemiology." When he examined water from the pump under his microscope, Dr. Snow described white particles which he couldn't explain. Cholera epidemics in England led to what became known as the Sanitary Movement led by a lawyer by the name of Edwin Chadwick. Although his idea was scientifically flawed because it was based on Galen's ancient theory of polluted air from decaying organic matter, the result was positive since it combatted the filth that accompanied the Industrial Revolution with its urbanization and overcrowding. Cholera epidemics profoundly altered social conditions so that by mid 19th century sanitation had become a matter of public interest. This eventually led to city planning (Paris), sewers and plumbing, parks and open spaces and the end result was better health -- indeed sanitation was far more important than scientific advances.

It wasn't until 1883 when Robert Koch, directing a German commission in Egypt and again the next year in Calcutta, isolated the bacteria which he called *Vibrio comma*. Everyone is vulnerable to cholera but the malnourished more so and although today it is easily treated with hydration and antibiotics, there continue to be several million cases worldwide each year, with more than 100,000 deaths -- mostly in Africa and India. There hasn't been an active case in this country for nearly a century, but in 2010 there was a severe outbreak in Haiti after a severe earthquake.

Typhoid was another common cause of lethal diarrhea or enteric fever. During the Civil War it was the leading cause of death because of unsanitary food preparation. No rat fleas or mosquitoes were necessary for transmission -- it was said that during the war "beans killed more than bullets." Everyone has heard of "Typhoid Mary" - Mary Mallon - who was an Irish cook for wealthy people in the New York City area. She frequently changed jobs, and names, and wherever Mary went, sickness (not sheep) was sure to follow -- some people died from it. Although Mary had no symptoms she was a carrier – presumably the reservoir was her gall bladder and she passed germs per rectum. She rarely washed her hands while cooking, believing that it wasn't necessary, and although she was told to stop cooking or to have her gall bladder removed she did neither and kept right on. In 1907 she was forcibly quarantined on North Brother Island in the East River near Riker's Island. But after three years Health Commissioner Lederle took pity and released her with the warning to find another profession. Once again Mary assumed aliases and for six more years kept doing what she knew best – and with the same result. She was tracked down again and was returned to the island where, after a total of 26 years in isolation, she died in 1932. Mary was a celebrity in her unique way, and to some people was a symbol of governmental undermining of individual liberties.

Although Typhus sounds like Typhoid it should be the other way around – typhoid sounds like typhus because the suffix "oid" imeans "like" – like typhus. However, the two diseases are NOT at all alike – they present differently and are due to different bugs. Earlier I mentioned Hans Zinsser's book *Rats, Lice and History* which he described as a "biography" of typhus. Typhus is caused by a Rickettsia which, like plague, is carried by rats -- but here it's not infected fleas that transmit the germ to man, but wingless mites or lice that don't fly but crawl – and bite. Body lice are prevalent in crowded, filthy places like prisons and concentration camps. Anne Frank died of typhus at Bergen Belsen and immediately after the war ended, survivors of Theresienstadt were almost wiped out by it. In 1892 an epidemic was traced to a single ship bearing Russian immigrants after a rough 28 day crossing. No one knew the cause except that it was brought in by those dirty Jewish immigrants so they all were rounded up and quarantined, most sent to Riverside Hospital on the same dismal North Brother Island where Typhoid Mary soon would be incarcerated.

Typhoid, typhus, cholera, yellow fever, small pox all stirred nativist fears about the nation's ethnic makeup and about the limitations of scientific medicine. Public health reforms began with increased scrutiny of the mental and physical health of arriving immigrants – keeping the sick out was imperative. Of far less concern was the effect of quarantine on those kept in enforced isolation. A 1947 novel by Albert Camus called *The Plague* described how forced quarantine during an epidemic of bubonic plague tore at the social fabric of a North African community and and now (September 2014) life is imitating fiction in West Africa where because of Ebola airlines are canceling flights, borders are closed, economies damaged, supplies dwindling and panic is taking hold.

The famous 1918 flu pandemic was due to a subtype of the influenza virus (H1Ni) which reemerged in 1976 as "Swine Flu" because its reservoir was in pigs. A few years later Swine Flu was followed by Bird Flu or Avian Flu (H5N1.) But what of some of the other pathogens that still endanger us? Measles is making a comeback although a vaccine developed in 1966 had virtually eliminated it – in fact, in 2000 measles was declared to have been eliminated in this country. Now, however, 10% of parents choose to delay or altogether skip their children's immunization shots because of misinformation about possible side effects, especially autism with the MMR vaccine against measles, mumps and rubella. So far this year there've been 16 outbreaks in this country with more than 560 cases, all related to non-vaccination. Measles can be lethal if there's no immunity – ask the Native Americans. WHO estimates that in the undeveloped world there are 14 deaths every *hour* in small children! There's no validity to the hysteria about autism which began in 1998 based on what turned out to be fraudulent claims of twelve cases reported to be due to the MMR vaccine. Numerous large epidemiological studies have failed to show any association but too many people believe what they want to believe.

Polio crested in the early 1950s, then declined dramatically when polio vaccines became available, but polio is not dead yet. Last year there were 24 reported cases in seven countries and so far this year that number has risen five fold to 117. When the Taliban forbade polio vaccinations and murdered dozens of health workers in Pakistan, the virus spread to neighboring Afghanistan and now India also is threatened. The Taliban claims that it's all a western plot to undermine Pakistan and parents are reminded that American intelligence faked a vaccination program in the search for Osama bin Laden. Should we worry? Its been suggested that failure to eradicate every case will cause the polio virus to proliferate wildly so that within a decade the whole world might be at risk again.

In 2003 SARS (severe acute respiratory syndrome) appeared in dozens of Asian countries and killed more than 700 people. Then in 2012 Middle East Respiratory Syndrome (MERS) appeared in twenty countries with about one third of more than 700 cases dying. SARS and MERS are due to coronaviruses which may be transmitted to man by infected bats and can be spread through the air human to human. In 1984 when AIDS was found to be due to HIV (human immunodeficiency virus) it was suggested that crossover from chimpanzees to man may have occurred in the early 20th century. The last naturally occurring case of anthrax in this country was in 1976, but this July the NYTimes reported that 75 lab workers at the CDC were accidentally exposed to anthrax spores. There's a very small risk for a similar accident with other infectious agents but this summer there were reports of lax safety standards at other labs. In 1978 a laboratory mishap spread virus to a ventilation system where it infected and killed a man and earlier this year, several vials of live small pox virus were found in an abandoned storage room at the NIH. And there continues to be debate about what to do with the last two known vials of small pox vaccine in the world? Should they be destroyed or saved to make vaccine?-- just in case.

The most common cause of acute gastroenteritis in this country is norovirus. The CDC estimates that each year it causes about 20 million illnesses, not just on cruise ships, and contributes to more than 50,000 hospitalizations and more than 500 deaths. Touching surfaces or objects contaminated with norovirus and then putting fingers to the mouth is all that it takes. A recent study found that within two to four hours after office workers touched a contaminated doorknob the virus could be detected in about 50%. By contrast, there were only about 20,000 confirmed cases of Lyme Disease last year, all contained within 13 states, but although we are told to check for tics after we walk in the woods, how many of us worry about touching doorknobs?

Let's not forget that the old "white plague" tuberculosis is still around. In 2012 about 2 billion people in the world were infected with nearly 9 million active cases and about 1.3 million deaths, second only to AIDS, at 1.6 million, the leading cause of death among infectious diseases. Moreover, multi drug-resistant TB is on the rise with around 500,000 new cases worldwide each year -- In the United States, out of about 10,000 cases of TB in 2012, only 83 were drug-resistant – still a very small number but it could rise. Responsibility for TB control is divided among more than 2,600 state and local agencies which is a recipe for inefficiency and cut-backs in funds for preventive programs. Most cases involve poor migrant workers, prisoners and AIDS patients and the homeless – none of whom have political lobbies arguing for them. Early in the 20th century health departments locked up patients with TB whose behavior posed a public health threat. Even after antibiotics became available, involuntary confinement was practiced and authorities still occasionally incarcerate patients who for whatever the reason won't take their medications. Usually it takes about two weeks after treatment is started before patients no longer are contagious.

Epidemics of plague and cholera may be past history but if bacteria or viruses mutate, they can develop renewed virulence or change their behavior. Everyone knows that because the influenza virus is constantly changing, each year vaccine manufacturers have to scramble to keep up. With airplane travel bad bugs from distant lands can cross the earth in hours rather than taking months in sailing ships so that an outbreak anywhere, is a risk everywhere, so there's no place for complacency. George Santayana's famous caveat that he who does not learn from the past is destined to relive it remains relevant so we might say that he who does not learn from the PEST (sorry, I couldn't resist) – or, from the history of plagues and pox – may suffer the consequences.

5. CHOLERA COMES TO PIERMONT

Farmer Nicholas Gesner (1765-1858) lived all of his life in Palisades, New York (then known as Rockland) which is three miles from my current home in Piermont. For most of his adult life Gesner recorded details of his daily activities in a journal which provided a fascinating picture of life in the area nearly two centuries ago. In 2015 a friend of mine, Alice Gerard, completed a fifty year preservation project of portions of the farmer's diary that originally was begun by her mother Alice Haagensen - still incomplete by the time she reached age 100. The result was four volumes, spanning 1829-1850, which I mined for material related to medical history and what I found was particularly interesting because it was written from a patient's perspective. What follows appeared in "South of the Mountains", the publication of The Historical Society of Rockland County (January-March, 2016.)

Three terse entries in Nicholas Gesner's diary revealed a long forgotten calamity that occurred in neighboring Piermont in 1849:

> Sept. 19: *Died at Piermont last Night 5 with Cholera and 12 Cases said And at Petersons (near Jerry) a Boarder died little before 12 to Day - a few Days Ago 2 also at Piermont.... Sickly in the place*
> Sept. 20: *The Cholera Rages at Piermont, 3 died last Night*
> Sept. 21: *It is said that 5 Deaths to Day at Piermont with Cholera.*

Cholera "raging." "Sickly in the place." At least fifteen deaths! Yet standard histories of Rockland County don't mention this event and the only acknowledgment was an obscure phrase contained in a booklet *Piermont. Three Centuries* (published in 1996 by The Friends of the

Piermont Public Library, p. 37) which noted that "church records refer to the number of church members who succumbed to cholera in 1849." No further detail. Surely this arcane subject was worth investigating.

From early times there were occasional outbreaks of smallpox, yellow fever and measles in Rockland County, but during the 19th century the most deadly scourge was cholera (see previous chapter). America's first epidemic of cholera began in June 1832 and by the end of that year, 3,515 people were dead in New York City out of a population of 250,000 (equivalent to more than 100,000 victims with today's population.) More than 40% were born in Ireland for as one intolerant physician wrote, "New York stands foremost as the grand focus and receptacle of the poverty and filth of Europe." People of means fled to the country. According to the *New York Evening Post*, "The roads, in all directions, were lined with well-filled stage coaches, livery coaches, private vehicles and equestrians, all panic-struck, fleeing the city, as we may suppose the inhabitants of Pompeii fled when the red lava showered down upon their homes."

Few medical men believed that cholera was contagious; most blamed the disease on miasmas (bad air) arising in poor neighborhoods. It was an era long before germ theory and the sanitation movement, a time when few bathed or washed, city streets were filthy, privies and drinking water drawn from polluted shallow wells, often located near seeping cesspools. Acute dehydration and electrolyte loss could cut a healthy person down within hours and quarantine methods did no good because cholera wasn't transmitted directly from person to person or by animal vectors. Medical treatment was the usual - bleeding, emetics, opiates - and it wasn't until the 1880s it was learned that cholera was due to a bacterial infection which spreads primarily through water fouled by human excrement usually ingested by eating unwashed fruits, vegetables or raw fish - indeed oysters from the Hudson were a favorite local delicacy. So the culprit wasn't bad air at all but bad water — the bacillus could live in water for long periods of time but once swallowed, and if it survived stomach juices, its toxin would play havoc with the intestinal tract.

On July 3, 1832 Nicholas Gesner noted in his diary, "Cholera in New York. People moved out this last week, hundreds. Some vessels have Stopped Running. Sorrowful time." That year more than 100,000 New Yorkers "eloped" to pure country air and, most likely, some fled up river which contributed to the spread to Rockland County. Gesner provided some more detail in the following entries:

July 6: *Many hundred families move from New York for to flee from the Asiatick Cholera. It began at Quebec and Montreal, crossed the Atlantic. It appears that it began there sometime in the first of January last.*
Aug. 31: *Cholera raged a few Days past in Closter. Several Died. Mrs. Bogert, in digging up her Sons cloths which were buried to wash them - she and a boy took it and both died. Cholera is now spread pretty much over all the United States. A Solemn Judgement* [by God upon sinful mankind.]
Sept. 1: *Robert Sneden poorly…with Bloody flux. Mrs. Chapman has Cholera in point.*
Sept 4: *Jacob Gesner's wife Betsy bad with Relax* [described elsewhere by NG as bloody and Slymy excrement.] *I got Away to go for Dr. Perry, little after 10 o'clock night. Dr. Perry came late in the night, intending to go to New York from Fort Lee and stopped and concluded that Betsy had the (Bloody) Dysentery.*
Sept. 7: Piercy preached excellent sermon, yea extraordinary. Good number hearers, suppose about 200 hearers. Many out doors. Text Amos: "prepare thyself to Meet thy God."
Sept 8: *A full house 8 or 10 Mourners…Oh! the tears, cries. The Lord present, we all on our knees praying to the Lord. Altho a mournful penitential time, yet what a Glorious time.*

The devout had little sympathy for the plight of the cholera-stricken poor. They believed the pestilence was due to poverty and sin - an angry "God's justice." Like with the flood and the plague of locusts, cholera was a means by which the Lord achieved moral purification and no wonder that church services were overflowing. Haverstraw's *North River Times* reported that one of the local victims Judge Cowen was "a man remarkable for his temperate habits and universally esteemed," but added that for every such estimable person affected, there were perhaps twenty more victims who are "addicted to habits of intemperance or uncleanliness and are swept off." Or, as *The Rockland County Messenger* put it, cholera is "chiefly confined to the vicious and filthy."

After the "plague" of 1832 abated sporadic cases recurred during the next two summers. On August 8, 1833 Gesner reported, "I was taken before Day-light this morning with Cholera Morbus." (This was a term then used for cases of acute gastroenteritis usually appearing in late summer.) Two days later he was "still vomiting and purging" but within another week reported, "I am considerably better. My appetite is better. I use circumspection." [?]

Then in 1849, after a seventeen year hiatus, epidemic cholera (then called Asiatic cholera) returned and, as Gesner described in his diary, this time Piermont felt the full force. In New York City that summer more than 5,000 died, many of their bodies buried in a mass grave on Randalls Island. In June ex-President James Polk, three months after leaving office, died of cholera. Two weeks later (July 3) his successor Zachary Taylor declared a day of national prayer for "public fasting, humiliation and prayer on account of the malignant disease." Exactly one year and one day after that, President Taylor, himself, developed symptoms of cholera - according to legend several hours after eating raw vegetables and a large bowl of unwashed cherries at the White House. He lasted five days and afterward his hearse was drawn by eight white horses with 100,000 people lining the funeral route. The fate of Piermont's victims that same year was scarcely noticed.

Except for Nicholas Gesner's observations, the only surviving primary source that documents any outbreak in Piermont in 1849 is a typewritten history of the First Baptist Church which suggested that something ominous was at work. It noted that three church elders died of cholera that summer: Brother John I. Wilne, age 41, Deacon Adrian Onderdonk, age 38, and Brother John Gahanna who while "administering to the wants of a large number of families afflicted with the cholera, was himself called to fall a victim to its fearful power in his 63rd year." How many more who were not church members were infected or died is unknown.

The next to last diary entry made by then 83 year old Nicholas Gesner was on July 20, 1850, but just two weeks later a far more reliable chronicler of local events, the *Rockland County Journal,* began publishing as a weekly newspaper. In the first issue the editor proclaimed that the paper would not indulge in "frivolous gossip" and vowed to provide "pungent, high-toned articles on the topics of the day" and so it was that five years later in 1854 when Piermont again was gripped by an outbreak of cholera, an unnamed reporter went over to see for himself and reported back in graphic detail.

> *RAVAGES OF THE CHOLERA IN PIERMONT*
> *It becomes our painful duty this week to record the existence beyond a doubt of Cholera in Piermont. During the last few days, the most*

exaggerated rumors have been in circulation and in order to arrive at the exact truth, we made a personal visit on Wednesday among all the dwellings in the infected district. Although, as we anticipated, the case was not as bad as rumor has made it. still, we witnessed scenes that would make the heart of a stoic ache. The first probably defined case of cholera was that of Timothy Driscoll who was taken on the 22d of July and died. On the last Sunday, Timothy Cronan on the hill, was taken and died the next day. The same night his little daughter, about ten years old was taken and also his wife who died on Tuesday. At the time of our visit, the little girl was laying on a heap of old bedding on the floor with no one to care for her or heed her wants. The flies literally fastened to her eyelids. As we looked on the pitiful scene we could not help wondering where the overseers of the poor were.... Up to Wednesday noon, eleven deaths had occurred from this cause and about twelve cases more were under treatment. The village Board of Trustees commenced the erection on Wednesday of a building to be used as a hospital selection for the site the ground near the river in the rear of Odd Fellows Hall [currently the Macedonian Baptist Church.] *It stands about 400 yards from any dwellings, and obviates the necessity of carrying the patients any great distance. There seems to be a complete panic especially among the railroad laborers, and those who have no families are leaving the place with as much haste as possible. It is our opinion that the disease is not contagious, and we hope for humanity's sake, the citizens of Piermont will not shun through fear their duty, especially toward the stricken.*

By the next week the situation had improved although there'd been two more deaths.

PROGRESS OF THE CHOLERA AT PIERMONT
Since our gloomy record last week of the ravages of the dreadful disease at Piermont, we have paid another visit, in company with Dr. Hopson, Physician of the Board of Health, [James A. Hopson was Piermont's first physician] *through the infected districts. Though we cannot, as we hoped, record this week the cessation of the frightful scourge, yet it has evidently reached its climax and a reasonable hope may be indulged that it will cease entirely. Were it in our power to convey an exact description of some of the scenes which actually occur*

> *during the prevalence of this pestilence, this would scarcely be credited. The idea of grappling with such a terrible visitor, surrounded with all the palliatives comforts which affection and wealth can throw around, is sufficiently terrifying but to see it in the abodes of the suffering poor, attended with want, destitution and desertion, is the very refinement of horror.*

The outbreak of 1854 wasn't as severe as those that began in 1832 and 1849 but this time southern and midwestern states also were hammered — more than 1,400 people died in Chicago alone. That same summer in London Dr. John Snow discovered that the cause of a cholera epidemic there came from drinking water from a single public pump. Also in 1854, the causative bacteria *vibrio cholerae* was isolated in Italy, but its full significance wouldn't be appreciated until the work of Louis Pasteur in France in the 1870s and Robert Koch in Germany during the 1880s.

Nicholas Gesner's scant observations in 1849 had established that a health crisis existed in nearby Piermont and because this transit hub seems to have been more effected than nearby inland towns, it seems likely that the water borne bacterium came from down river. At mid-19th century the village was going through a growth spurt with its population swelling to more than 2,000, many of them unmarried Irish railroad workers who were living in hastily constructed unsanitary quarters along the polluted *Slote* — outhouses emptied directly into the creek where, no doubt, the workers washed themselves and their clothes. A booster writing to the *Rockland County Journal* (June 19, 1852) praised many new developments in the village, but described "shanties which will very soon be torn down and a neat row of cottages will supply their place."

Living conditions were harsh for the thousands of Irish railway workers who fled the potato famine at home during the 1840s to seek refuge in America. The workers frequently were exploited and abused by unscrupulous contractors and sometimes this led to violent riots which fueled nativist perceptions of the Irish as a rowdy and disorderly group. Context for what might have prevailed in Piermont can be appreciated by a tragedy which occurred in Malvern, Pennsylvania in 1832 where fifty-seven recently arrived Irish railroad workers died of cholera. Cramped living conditions helped to rapidly spread the disease through the work crew; those who didn't succumb tried to seek aid from the larger community but were shunned. Fear of the spread of cholera with rising anti-Irish and anti-Catholic sentiment in the wake of increased immigration created a situation in which these laborers were forced to suffer without any medical relief. It was as if they were an expendable race apart. The fifty-seven men who died in Malvern were hastily buried in a mass grave along the tracks on which they labored.

During the 1850s, Piermont was the busiest railroad terminal in the country; huge supplies of strawberries, dairy products, livestock, lumber and steel shipped 26 miles downstream to a terminal on Duane Street. Roughly ninety acres of land along the river bank, created from crushed Palisades rock and landfill, were crammed with terminal buildings, depots, two roundhouses that could accommodate 30 locomotives, a hotel, livery stables, repair shops, markets and dry goods stores. Conditions were chaotic with incessant din from clanging anvils, steamboat and locomotive whistles and smoke from engines and furnaces filled the air.

In 1841, six months after the first section of the Erie Railroad opened from Piermont to Ramapo, the company was in bankruptcy and the workers were restless; as one report described "Irish work gangs brawled among themselves or with smaller groups of Germans in drunken fist fights and rioting." The railroad's fortunes fluctuated and in 1857, when its affairs again were in critical condition, a general reduction of wages was put into effect; 250 freight handlers in Piermont had their pay reduced from $1 to 95 cents for an eleven hour day. When the men learned that the president of the line would not take a reduction in his $25,000 annual earnings, they went on strike and everything ground to a halt — in four days 200 carloads of produce backed up. In order to protect the property and disperse the strikers, the sheriff of Rockland called for the Piermont Guard who turned out with fixed bayonets and ammunition. When 100 immigrant "scabs" escorted by 25 policemen arrived by boat from New York City to replace the strikers they were driven off with some thrown in the river, but eventually the strikers were subdued and relative calm restored. In this tinder box, sanitation surely was not a high priority and unclean conditions were conducive for an outbreak of cholera and if wealthy people who lived high in the surrounding hills were less ravaged, it was not because of any superior morality but because their drinking water was less likely to be contaminated.

Published histories about Piermont at mid-19th century emphasize contributions of civic leaders, completion of the new pier out into the Hudson River, incorporation and renaming the village, and the great day

(May 14, 1851) when President Millard Fillmore, Secretary of State Daniel Webster and more than three hundred notables rode the first passenger train from Piermont to Lake Erie. However, the few existing primary sources from those years suggest a darker alternative narrative. Nicholas Gesner's diary and the local church records from 1849 and the journalist's eye witness accounts in 1854 employed such terms as frightful scourge, suffering poor, panic among railway workers, shanties, destitution and desertion, deaths of church elders who tried to help, need for a cholera hospital. Although some of this may have been overwrought, clearly, everything was not celebration and prosperity during Piermont's glory years. Nevertheless, later writers of local history seem to have preferred emphasizing triumph to tragedy.

On August 19, 1854, one week after his second visit to Piermont, the same reporter for the *Rockland County Journal* reflected on what he'd witnessed and bitterly criticized the wealthy class who in his judgment had distanced themselves from poor victims:

> *They never enter the cabin of the afflicted lest their garments should be soiled or their reputations in certain circles depreciated. They can scarcely pass within a hundred yards of the abode of pestilence and poverty without turning up their dainty noses...and that is one train of thought suggested by Our visits through the cholera districts of Piermont.*

Nothing more appeared in print about cholera outbreaks in Piermont either in 1849 or 1854 and the actual number of victims, especially among anonymous railroad workers, was never recorded. No doubt some good souls tried to help and many years later (February 5, 1887) the *Rockland County Journal* reported the following:

> *Dr. James A. Hopson, whose funeral was held last Saturday, was a resident of this village for many years, and at one time was the leading physician in our county; but through misfortune, for the past ten years his practice was very limited. During the cholera epidemic of 1849 he was of great assistance to the poor people of this town, and although he has not practiced of any account for the past few years, he will be missed by a great many who used to see him pass their door daily. The Doctor died of softening of the brain.*

Lacking additional primary source material we can only speculate about the magnitude of devastation wrought by cholera in Piermont at mid-19th century. Nevertheless, any fair description of the village's history should be sensitive to the plight of ordinary people even as the contributions of civic leaders are celebrated.

6. LOVE LETTERS OF A COUNTRY DOCTOR

Nicholas Gesner's journal described medical matters in 19th century Rockland County from a patient's perspective, but not long afterward, a physician's perspective was provided in a most unusual format - love letters! Versions of this and the next essay appeared in earlier Meanderings and what follows here was published in the winter 2017 issue of the Rockland County Historical Society's "South of the Mountains."

In 1997 Jeanne DuBois Crawford became aware that her mother Ruth Dingman Crawford had discovered a trove of some 400 "courtship letters" that Jeanne's grandparents, Clarence Dingman and Louise Berry had exchanged between 1898 and 1908. Most were written during an extended period when Louise was living in Minneapolis while Clarence was a struggling young doctor in Spring Valley, NY. The letters were published by Ms. Crawford in 2009 and amidst expressions of longing for Louise, Clarence's letters contained numerous vignettes which depicted the stress and occasional discouragement of a country doctor working in relative isolation.

In 1904 John Clarence Dingman (1881-1971) took over the medical practice of his ailing father who had come to rural Spring Valley, N.Y. in 1876. In those days one could enter medical school straight out of high school and in 1904 both Clarence and his brother Alva completed the two year course of studies at Columbia's College of Physicians and Surgeons. Office hours were held three times a day in his home office and the rest of the day (and night) was for house calls. Clarence ground his own medicines with a mortar and pestle and, often as not, was paid in goods instead of cash. There were few telephones and the customary way of summoning the doctor was to rap on his door. His early career saw the advent of the automobile, but frequent flat tires, breakdowns and treacherous roads made traditional conveyances more reliable in bad weather – e.g. horse drawn sleigh, even snowshoes. But all wasn't stressful or gloomy and Clarence Dingman sometimes described moments of exhilaration about the beauty of nature as he made his lengthy circuits.

The following are selections from the letters of a conscientious and compassionate physician who was blessed with a poetic soul:

> *A real blizzard is in progress without...I had the pleasure of contending with the elements the whole afternoon and I was very glad to reach home again. Had it not been for the storm I would now be on the road for Pearl River where a pneumonia patient is awaiting. But the storm is too severe and as they have plenty of medicine and advice already, I will wait until tomorrow. (January 4, 1905)*

> *I have been called out the last three nights and have been in bed just six hours during the last two nights. Night before last about midnight, I was called to see a man in Monsey who was taken suddenly ill with great pain. Well, I did all that I could do for him and then took him up to the Suffern Hospital where we operated upon him. When I reached home at about eight o'clock the next morning, I was pretty nearly done for – not from loss of sleep but from the nervous strain and responsibility. (October 16, 1905)*

> *It seems to me that the life to live is one in a country...unhampered by the demands and restrictions of our crowded civilization. It emphasizes all the more forcibly that the farther one gets away from nature, the harder it is to live a true life. I am all the more thankful that my lot is cast in the country, and among a comparatively simple people. (September 20, 1907)*

> *I have had some very sick people this week. Sometimes, I feel as if the responsibility would be too much for me and I have to tell myself not to care about results but to go ahead and do the best I can. One man...died here Friday night. He was only thirty-seven and had such*

a promising future it seemed hard not to be able to do anything for him. (November 25, 1907)

I might be able to do some good this afternoon for there is a little two year old boy waiting for me to take off his plaster jacket and put on a new one. And then there is an old man who has been sick a few days and yesterday I found him fully convinced that he was going to die and consequently was much worse. It took me some time to convince him that he was going to get better and in order to do so he must believe that he was. (January 8, 1908)

Most of my work is out in the country and that means long drives over rough roads. Yesterday I sat in a wagon all day long until ten last night – probably thirty-five miles in all. It was fearfully muddy and I was a sight. Until today when it has snowed and rained the weather has been splendid for some time.... This is indeed God's country... it was beautiful. Snow clad hills in every direction. ...The world is so beautiful and it is so wonderful to live and the possibilities are so great...((March 7, 1908)

I had a bad day yesterday. Everything seemed to go wrong. Had some very sick people and everything seemed to go to delay me until I became nervous and irritable which only made matters worse.... I had a long twenty mile trip to make and couldn't seem to get away from the village. Had sent for a nurse for a sick patient and she didn't show up and I was afraid to leave the patient until she did. Well at last she did and I finally started...Once out of the country in sight of the dear old hills I felt better at once and quite enjoyed the long drive home behind the team. (March 9, 1908)

I am dog tired.... I have had only six hours sleep since Monday morning and since then have driven over eighty miles of muddy roads and have made over forty sick calls, not counting office patients, you might imagine how tired I am tonight. (March 12, 1908)

I have had a very, very busy week and am pretty well played out. Mud! Mud!

Mud! Nothing but mud — and such mud! The wagon wheels sink in up to the hubs and the poor ponies have a hard time of it. I come in every time almost covered with it and we have even had chocolate pudding for dessert twice this week! (March 16, 1908)

After a visit to a twenty year old "young Jew" dying of tuberculosis: *Four weeks ago he became worse and since then his mother has not been able to leave him so their only means of support is the sister – who makes four dollars per week.... I wormed out of him that they had only three dollars left and owed the grocer six. His mother is exhausted and sick from loss of sleep and the poor chap has been fighting for breath for a good many days. When I told him that I would take care of him and to have the medicines charged to me at the druggist, and that I would see that he was supplied with milk and eggs, his gratitude was pathetic. "Doctor" he said, "if I ever get out of this I will pay you back if I have to wash your feet. I never expected to hear such words from a doctor." (March 30, 1908)*

We sometimes think that our problems are overwhelming and are going to be too much for us, but what are they to the trials and sufferings of so many? It makes me feel like thirty cents, after I have been feeling blue and discouraged and have wondered if it were of any use to try any longer, to find some poor chap contending with a brave face against odds compared with which my troubles are like those of a spoiled child crying for candy. (March 30, 1908)

While returning from a trip to the nearest garage in Paterson, NJ, there was a mishap:

On the way home my supply of acetylene gas gave out and we were forced to come most of the way home with only the oil lamps. Just below Monsey although I was driving carefully, we crashed into the rear of a huge market truck loaded with empty barrels. We all narrowly escaped being cut by the flying glass from the front glass front which was shattered. The whole front of the car was crushed - lamps, bonnet, etc., although the engine and driving mechanism was injured and we came the rest of the way under the car's own power....[The next morning] drove what was left of the car back to Paterson. It will *cost me about $75 to have it repaired and it almost makes me sick to think of it. (April 4, 1908)*

A call has just come to see a little baby who has been worrying me for some days. He is a dear little fellow, only six months old, and so friendly. It is a case of advanced summer diarrhea and he has been sick some weeks already. (July 27, 1908)

Have just seen that baby again. It is quite critically ill, but is no worse tonight than this morning. I have hopes of pulling it through but my heart fails me. It is such a dear baby and I fairly love it. I am going to ask God tonight when I pray to save that baby. (July 28, 1908) Everything seems to go wrong this morning. That little baby is dying. (July 31, 1908)

I have had to drive the horse today and aside from the slowness, have rather enjoyed it. It is so beautiful tonight. There is a beautiful full moon and the air is so cool and fresh... The stars were shining, although dimmed by the splendor of the young moon. (August 4, 1908)

I was late in getting back last night...what pitiful things I saw. It is a little family, just a couple and their three year old child. The wife has been a patient of mine for years. She is inclined to melancholia and some time ago became an atheist. She reads loads of cheap, lurid novels and for some time has believed that everyone in town was busy saying bad things about her. Last night I found her with her husband and two other men holding her in bed, a raving, mad woman. Her strength was almost super human and her cries were pitiful – seemed to be afraid that someone was going to knife her and then she lapsed into a lot of cheap novel phrases about a rich man trying to ruin her and get her to leave her husband. It was so pitiful and, at the same time, so sordid. Genuine, legitimate grief and suffering is often unavoidable, but it seems so strange that a woman would deliberately bring herself to this condition. I stayed until she was somewhat quieter and came away. (August 21, 1908)

> *I have been just a little blue and discouraged about my work lately. I have been so rushed that I allowed the office to become very untidy and poorly equipped. My memory too, becomes overcrowded at times and something is continually slipping. I am starting a system of cards for recording cases, so that I will not have to tax my memory so much. (August 27, 1908)*
>
> *Spent quite a busy evening in the office with patients. Went out once to quiet a hysterical school teacher. She was sobbing as though her heart would break, but I held her hand and petted her until she quieted down – plain case of overwork. (November 16, 1908)*

John Clarence Dingman practiced in Spring Valley for many years and when he died at age 90 in 1971 a colleague remembered him as "the dean of Rockland County medical practitioners."

7. DANCE CLASS

From time immemorial medical students had more than academics on their minds and 400 young men who attended the Rutgers Medical College in Lower Manhattan between 1826 and 1830 were no exceptions. Many of them came from rural backgrounds and were exposed to temptations in Olde New York that they'd never experienced back home. What follows here are descriptions of the extra-curricular activities of two high-spirited country bumpkins as extracted from their correspondence or diary entries.

John Rosencrantz of Ho-Ho-Kus, NJ attended two terms at Rutgers Medical College (1826-1827 and 1827-1828) and received an honorary medical degree in 1830. **Asa Fitch** of Salem, NY (forty miles from Albany) attended only the 1828-1829 term. Both students were born in 1809 and being the sons of country doctors followed in their father's footsteps, albeit with little enthusiasm. As we shall see, although each of them practiced medicine briefly after obtaining their licenses, both abandoned the profession as soon as opportunity permitted.

Elijah Rosencrantz was one of the few doctors in rural Bergen County during the early 19th century. When his oldest son John was fifteen he was sent to pursue "liberal studies" at an academy that probably was located in New York City. However, because of financial pressure, there was a change of plans and the ailing and aging father reluctantly arranged for his son to enter the family business. Early letters to siblings and friends had described squirrel hunting, sleighing and hunting, suggesting that John was more a typical teenager than a serious scholar; his brother once complained, "we can scarce read your writing." And when his son entered Rutgers medical school, Elijah's letters were filled with paternal advice to be respectful of elders, avoid bad company and to write home frequently:

I wish you my son to apply yourself to your studies, take necessary exercise and amusement but let them not intrude on your hours of study.... The many inducements to take you from your studies by the practice and customs of the young people in this country give me some anxiety for fear you will give away too much...Exercise and some company is necessary to become acquainted with the world, but I shall still hope that you will not give yourself too much to the pleasures and diversions of customs of this place. It is impossible to apply the mind to study when it is continually intoxicated with the idea of company and those bewitching frolics common to this country. You will not disappoint me I hope of keeping yourself and your desires of company and pleasures of youth under due restraint. (January 30, 1825)

For emphasis, four days later, Elijah wrote again:

Your main object should be knowledge of your intended profession and secondly knowledge of the world which are both indispensably necessary to your becoming useful to yourself and society... The field before you is great. Great industry and perseverance is necessary to make your reputation in your profession. This I trust you are sensible of and will not disappoint me. (February 3, 1827)

At the beginning of John Rosencrantz's second term at Rutgers his father made an uncharacteristic concession:

I had thought to have mentioned it to you before you left home that if you had any wish to go to a dancing school this winter, I would have no objection provided it be respectable and not too expensive, but this you must keep to yourself, let it not be known here. If it be your wish you may let me know directly and the terms. I do it to meet your wish only, it may be an accomplishment. (November 7, 1826)

Only fragments of their later correspondence still exist, so it's not known whether or not John took advantage of his father's offer. However, the following year **Asa Fitch** was more descriptive in his diary. From age

12 until his death at age 70, Asa recorded mundane details of his personal life in journals, including the four month period during the winter of 1828-29 when he travelled from his upstate home to New York City to study at Rutgers Medical College

Asa Fitch was a virtuous farm boy and had a strict upbringing; as a teenager he scolded himself, "I must not idle away my time…. I must do better. I *mus*t do better." Although he showed aptitude for botany and geology, both his father of the same name and his grandfather were physicians and wished him to enter the family vocation. So after graduation from high school, Asa was apprenticed to a local physician and that winter entered the Vermont Academy of Medicine. Originally called Castleton Medical Academy, it was the first independent medical school in New England. After completing a term in Vermont, Asa chastised himself about his insufficient application to study: "I regret I have not learned more. I have often been too inattentive, and have heard whole lectures, without remembering scarcely an idea which they contained. It is now… too late to repent, and I must make amends in my future application." Opportunity for self-improvement came the next winter when he enrolled for a term of lectures and surgical demonstrations at the Rutgers Medical College in lower Manhattan (now Tribeca.)

Most of the entries in Asa Fitch's journal described attractions and temptations of city life: how he walked wide-eyed along Broadway, the Bowery and Greenwich Village; how he ferried across the East River to visit the Brooklyn Navy Yard; how whenever a fire bell rang out he'd dash off after the engines to watch the show; museums and theater provided entertainment and he often attended book auctions. His strict religious background was tested as he visited various churches, seemingly more out of curiosity than religious fervor.

Undoubtedly the highlight of Asa's social life in New York, which occupied a major portion of his journals, were dancing classes for men that were given in a hall in the 11th Ward, a rowdy section noted for its multitude of beer saloons. At first he was shy and clumsy but diligently practiced the steps in his room at night after it was too dark to read or write. After twenty-three lessons, he became self-confident and comfortable in "gallanting" the young ladies at cotillions. He learned to bow and shake hands according to current etiquette and he mastered the "art of conversation." After all, "The profession I have chosen requires an ability to conduct myself in all grades of society with ease and propriety." Also, he was beguiled by young women, although with some reservations:

> *Previously, I'd delighted to look on beautiful features and to contemplate the fair sex with admiration [but] my natural diffidence and bashfulness forbade my forming any acquaintance except when circumstances made it unavoidable…[but] New York is no place for [feminine] beauty. All the paraphernalia of art will never supplant this defect. I have not since I arrived here, seen looks so fascinating to me, as those of the country fair ones, where the tyrant fashion has not so [held] sway.*

On Christmas Eve Asa was homesick and, longing for companionship, went partying with a few like-minded friends. They drank hot whiskey punch, Holland gin cocktails and cognac slings and before long the giddy group was full of "life and animation…felt a glow of thought…[and their conversation was] frivolous and risable." The drunken students stumbled through their dance routines, sang off-tune and staggered home very late. Inevitably, this was followed by morning-after sickness, self-recrimination and vows not to repeat the debauch – at least not for a few days.

Asa Fitch's four months in lower Manhattan was the longest time he'd ever been away from home and by the end of February he was eager to return to Salem. Before leaving he purchased a medical bag, lancets, chemicals and books and as the end of the term approached, he was pleased that he'd made "rapid strides toward the age of manhood." On his last night he put on his finery and his "blackened and shining boots," resolved that "this shall be the happiest, sweetest, liveliest evening I have yet known in New York. I will let out one notch." At the cotillion, while changing to his dancing pumps, he mused:

> *When shall I wear them again? I know not, but hope the folks in Salem do not think dancing the awful thing which they have for a few years past. Where is the harm in dancing? I have not yet found it out. I have not yet experienced the least ill consequence from it. Nor does my conscience tell me it's wrong or sinful."…. I have now come to a room where many an evening for the last three months I have witnessed the manners and customs of city life, the gayety and frivolity – where many an hour has been passed "treading the steps of the giddy dance,*

> *on the light fantastic toe." Ah, they were happy hours – hours of enjoyment. And with this evening they terminate forever.*

That night Asa led some of the quadrilles, proudly holding his head "as straight and stiff as a dandy." He knew that when he returned to his sober rural community both family and church leaders would reprimand him for frivolous behavior, especially his dancing but he had no regrets. Undaunted, he had derived great pleasure from the manners and customs of city life and vowed never to return to "say-nothing-to-nobody-ness"; never again to be an "ill-bred booby."

> *I am not prepared to renounce it [dancing]...my determination at the outset was to rid myself of the extreme diffidence, timidity, tongue-tiedness...This would never do for me when I was a doctor...I was resolved to cure myself of it.... I can now go into company, yes, polite company, and feel myself at home...I have danced, I have played, I have kissed rosy cheeks, I have won maidens' smiles. Yet I do not think I have gone astray, or opened the wounds of my Saviour... or sinned against my God.... And if dancing is to be condemned from the vicious habits to which it leads, I can aver that I have not felt this tendency. I have not gambled. I have not squandered away money. I have had no illicit connections. I have not even had any such inclinations. Never, no never.*

After his winter sojourn at Rutgers Medical Ciollege, Asa Fitch returned to Salem and apprenticed again with a local doctor. In August 1828 he returned to Castleton as an advanced student and attended the same lectures as during his first term there. Naturally, life in Vermont was not comparable to what he'd experienced in New York. He dutifully attended church services, participated in the debating society and sought opportunities to meet young ladies; the highlight of the year was the arrival of a "caravan of animals" – a traveling circus. But he was restless and eager to strike out on his own: "Oh, may it ever be my lot to be contented – to be happy, in whatever sphere I may be placed, nor pine away my life, with needless gloomy thoughts, when at best there is sorrow enough." Having completed a second course of lectures at the Vermont Academy and receiving credit for his studies at Rutgers, Asa had to defend his dissertation, "Natural Sciences and Their Importance to Medicine" and then pass a three hour oral examination. Finally, with diploma and medical license in hand, he married a local girl, "attracted more by her mind than her beauty." He practiced in her hometown of Stillwater for six years, but his various experiences left Asa with a "cordial distaste" for the life of a country doctor; he regarded himself as too honest to compete with the quacks and charlatans in the profession because of his resolve to give medicine only when needed and only in necessary doses.

In truth, Asa Fitch's passion always had been for -- insects! Since early childhood he habitually crawled around on hands and knees collecting all manner of creeping things in his "bug net." Neighbors called him "The Bug Catcher." In 1838 he gave up medical practice for good, returned to Salem to attend his ailing father's business and remained on the family's 600 acre farm for the remainder of his life. In 1855 he was appointed as New York State's first professional entomologist and, in time, was recognized as America's leading authority, his fourteen voluminous reports "The Noxious and Other Insects of New York State," recognized as classics in the field.

John Rosencrantz assisted his father in his medical practice until Elijah died in 1832. In a letter to a younger brother, John complained of "the dull monotony of life…[how] unrelenting routine is one of the greatest antidotes to sentiment and the busy imagination of youth…There is no room for fancy in the reality of this world." Nor was there time for dancing. Indeed, much of his time was taken with getting paid for his travail. He described how "the people around here are an infernal set with few exceptions. They don't care to pay bills. We must call for it [even] if it is five miles – earning it twice."

> *Although I am the son of a country physician and brought up in the country, yet I know no more of the life and the perplexities of one who practices here and lives by it, then a new born babe….*[in a postscript] *It is a Monday morning and I have just come in and have not a cent… Hell and dander – I wish the profession was in oblivion.*

A few years after his father died, John Rosencrantz gave up medical practice and moved to Philadelphia where he worked for the large Ripka textile mills. He married the owner's daughter, and since there were no other young males in the family, he became involved in running the Ripka business and never looked back.

Asa Fitch's medical career also was short-lived and undistinguished but he went on to achieve distinction as a prime mover in developing entomology as a profession in America. But both young men's writing provided a vivid description of student life early in the 19th century and although each of them went on to lead successful non-medical careers, it's fair to presume that neither regretted the frolics of their student days. Their eyes had been opened to new delights and, no doubt, dancing days and nights in Manhattan were among their fondest memories.

8. HYSTERIA AND HOLMES AT DARTMOUTH

I discussed a different perspective on 19th century medical education at a meeting of The Medical History Society of New Jersey in New Brunswick, NJ.

When Dartmouth Medical School (then called the New Hampshire Medical Institute) began offering a medical degree in 1812, all candidates had to attend two full courses of lectures, possess a competent knowledge of Latin, "sustain a good moral character" and write a dissertation on a subject of their choice "which he may be called on to read and defend at his examination as the Faculty may direct." Thesis topics selected by more than 1,200 students between 1815 and 1881 mainly concerned mundane subjects, especially infectious diseases which were the leading causes of sickness and death. Less common topics included animal magnetism, tight lacing, masturbation, intemperance in eating, suspended animation, bloodletting and miasma.

What follows next are selections from four student dissertations that were written respectively by Otis Ayer (1841), Henry B. Tibbetts (1845), Charles H. Fischer (1847) and George Page (1852), each addressing the subject of Hysteria. Considered together, they reflect the prevailing confusion about the nature of this perplexing condition. As one frustrated clinician of the time complained, hysteria could present in "a thousand different forms and we cannot grasp any of them." Symptoms enumerated in the theses included choking (globus hystericus), palpitations, seizures, anesthesia, contortions, flatulence, somnambulism and such behavioral oddities as excess talking, uncontrolled laughing, weeping, screaming, capriciousness, seductiveness, nymphomania and predilection for drama.

The full pharmacopeia of 19th century medicine was employed with variable success: strychnine, arsenic, cinchona, laudanum, valerian, zinc, tonics, cathartics, enemas, emetics and bleeding by lancet, cup or leech. One of the students wrote that "cold water is almost a specific, applied as a bath or by sprinkling or cold douche…cold water will scarcely fail of accomplishing its object if vigorously applied." (To be sure, vigor was required for all forms of "heroic" treatment.)

These four Dartmouth students could scarcely have been aware that they were in the midst of a profound transformation of medical thinking. The ancient humoral theories and "systems" which dominated medicine from the time of Hippocrates and Galen were becoming obsolete. Indeed the school's catalogue in 1847 noted that those lectures devoted to Theory and Practice were "mainly intended to guide the student in the acquisition of Truth and not Doctrine":

> *It is deemed unnecessary to examine, historically or critically, the great Medical theories of the past or present time, or to attempt the enlistment of the feelings or the judgment in condemning or upholding more abstract opinions.… All elaborate exposition of mere hypothesis is sedulously avoided and every effort made to give an intelligible history of those diseases which the practitioner is most likely to encounter.*

Such a statement couldn't have been made a half century earlier, but during the early 19th century a generation of young American medical students were travelling to Paris, as if to Mecca, in order to be enlightened. A main attraction was the abundance of cadavers, more than 4,000 a year, to practice their dissecting skills upon; not only were bodies cheap and available (a cadaver could be purchased for only thirty sous), so were wine and women. In post-Revolutionary France the notion took hold that the human body answered the same laws as the rest of the physical universe. It was the dawn of bedside teaching where a doctor learned to directly observe, record, and later correlate and classify. Moreover, proof could be found by looking inside for as Xavier Bichat famously explained in *Anatomie generale* (1801), a physician could spend twenty years taking bedside notes on obscure outward signs of diseases but "open a few corpses, and immediately this obscurity, which observation alone would never have revealed, will disappear."

Concerning hysteria, an emerging theme was that correlation of anatomical and clinical observations eventually would disclose a tangible explanation for the condition. Of course, none of our four earnest neophytes had any direct experience in patient care yet and relied almost entirely on their hastily scribbled lecture notes or reading textbooks in Dartmouth's well stocked library, which during the 1840s contained more than one thousand volumes. Perhaps they'd read the French physician Louyer-Villermay who asserted that hysteria could be attributed to such things as "an ardent and lascivious uterine system...voluntary or forced continence, sometimes onanism...a burning imagination...an overly tender or excitable heart..overuse of perfumes...reading novels." And surely they were familiar with the recently published lectures of Sir Thomas Watson who acknowledged that although "dysfunction of the uterus and its appendages may be mediated by the nervous system, how they do so we no more know than we know how the little finger is bent when we resolve to bend it."

The introduction of the dissertation that was written by Dartmouth senior Charles Fischer (Windham County, Connecticut) stood out for its sheer verbosity:

> *Among the varied and complicated "ills which flesh is heir to," there is not one, probably in the whole catalogue, so infinitely varied, as that Protean Malady, which forms the subject of this present Dissertation; neither is there one which demands from us more sympathy for its victims, including alike the suffering patient and the...baffled practitioner, occupying as it does a front rank in the list of frequent diseases, affecting mostly the active, the ardent and the intelligent, those of warm hearts and generous impulses, existing alike in count and in town, including the landmarks of time, overlapping the boundaries of Princes and Kings and Nations, appearing in all countries and under all climates, existing under all circumstances, and in every possible variety of form and of feature, confined exclusively to neither sex, exempting neither wealth nor rank nor station, is still maintained, as it has done from "time immemorial," its tyrannous supremacy; defying with almost absolute impunity, the investigations of science and the Therapia of Arts.*

Yes, that was a single run-on sentence! But his classmate Otis Ayer (New Hampton, New Hampshire) got straight to the point emphasizing that hysteria was a legitimate entity:

> *Among the diseases which manifest a partiality for the female sex, Hysteria holds a prominent station. It is a disease, the nature of which there was formerly little known, It has been viewed by our remote predecessors as a trifling affair made up of nervousness, fancifulness, and imbecility; not infrequently it has scarcely been treated with common humanity – often turned into a ridicule and considered as undeserving serious attention…Every filthy and disgusting odor, and every abominable drug that the surface or bowels of the earth affords has been unsparingly used in its cure. But happy for the unfortunate patient, as well as creditable to the profession, observation and investigation have cast new light…. Now instead of its being looked upon as a combination of nervousness, fancifulness and hallucination which associate for the purpose of tormenting the gentler sex, it is divested of its ghostly character, has assumed a tangible form and become subject to fixed pathological laws. Hysteria is a disease which varies in severity from the slightest abaration [sic] from health to a malady the most annoying to the patient and baffling to the physician of any which the human system is susceptible.*

Otis Ayer noted further that the pathology of hysteria, "although not so well known as in many other diseases…yet is generally admitted to be confined to the uterus and its appendages… [Some] have advanced the opinion that spinal irritation is the immediate cause….[and] claim that by applying appropriate treatment to the spine, the symptoms will disappear or be mitigated -- but it has been the misfortune of others to be called to treat cases that would not yield to such remedies." As for treatment, Ayer wrote that "depended upon individual circumstances – if the patient is plethoric bleed her occasionally…if debilitated, recommend a generous diet, purgatives, exercise and cheerful company."

Writing four years later, Henry Tibbets (Northfield, Massachusetts) cautioned that traditional theory concerning a uterine cause might be insufficient:

Hysteria, though not exclusively, is chiefly confined to the female sex. The range of its sway is almost entirely confined to the period which intervenes between the commencement and the complete cessation of the uterine functions.... There is something peculiar in the female organization which renders them especially the subjects of this remarkable affliction. From all the circumstances relating to the peculiarities of the disease it may be inferred that the proximate causes of hysteria are seated in the uterus and its appendages, a doctrine which is indeed expressly implied in the name given to this affliction..... The idea that the uterus was the seat as well as sole cause of the hysteric passion is as old as the times of Hippocrates and Galen and seems to have descended from generation to generation like some ancient heirloom so that even in these days, when an enlightened pathological knowledge has proved its fallacy, there are not wanting those who still insist on clinging to the ancient theory that hysteria arises from derangements of genital function in a vast majority of cases, will readily be admitted but that its "seat" and whole existence is in the uterus" is a position which cannot be sustained, when we know that hysteria may exist without any previous or present abnormal condition of the uterus or its appendages, and that every variety of uterine disease may exist any length of time without inducing hysteria

Henry Tibbets went on to speculate vaguely about the action of a "ganglionic reflex" located somewhere in the spinal cord that worked mysteriously, comparable to why when we see some one yawn, we "give way to the inclination" and mimic it.

Writing last, George Page (Haverhill, New Hampshire) rejected the uterine theory outright and understood that the culprit was "the mind and its influences." He suggested that in addition to some nervous system pathology, cultural factors may account for the marked prevalence in women which needed to be addressed:

That hysteria is a disease of the nervous system and not of the uterus simply, we think may be shown beyond a doubt. From the name it appears absurd to apply the same to any condition with which it may meet in the male, but this error must be attributable to the older writer, for the same excitable condition of the nervous system does occasionally present itself in males as is attested by good observers. The different systems of education of the sexes accounts in a great measure for the frequency with which the disease is met in the females over that of the male. Boys are sent at an early age to school where the greater share of their time is spent in outdoor exercise -- running, jumping, leaping, while the girls, like tender plants, by nature of much more fragile constitutions, are kept in heated rooms without being permitted to breathe the fresh air…Thus they acquire a precocity of mental development at the expense of the physical. So this method of bringing up the children must be ascribed as a reason for the difference in bodily health of the sexes, the development of the muscular and nervous systems of the young men… In no disease is it more important that the mind should be operated upon by proper influences than in hysteria. If the disease seems to have originated In, or to be dependent upon loss of friends, or disappointment in some love affair, the patient's circumstances should if possible be completely changed, less attention [paid] to her own condition, and her interest enlisted in matters of general interest. In this way often times much more good may be done than by dosing in medicines… No more agreeable and certain mode of accomplishing this can be advised than journeying or taking a voyage to a foreign country, but if the circumstances of the patient do not allow of this expense, her habits of life at home must be completely changed and her time occupied in some healthful and interesting pursuit.

Concerning this last suggestion, Henry Tibbetts had an interesting alternative treatment: "If the person [is] in any degree predisposed to this affection, early and judicious marriage." To be sure this wasn't a new idea for more than two millennia earlier Hippocrates wrote, "I advise maidens who suffer from hysteria to marry as soon as possible. For if they conceive, they will be cured." Charles Fischer agreed that a patient's life style is significant, and was pleased to note that "the progress of science" was abolishing superstition:

A great majority of cases of hysteria are the results of an improper mode of life and the disease might have been obviated by a change in that mode. All of the exciting causes of hysteria should be avoided, especially by females…late hours, strong mental excitement, excessive sexual indulgence…in short, all of the thousand and one modes of dissipation and excess attendant on the routine of an easy and luxurious life. Active physical exercise should be resorted to -- riding on horseback, walking, sailing and all the various gymnastic exercises. If scheming mammas and "pennywise" dummas were more considerate, if to be delicate and "beautifully weak" was not deemed a necessary accomplishment in fashionable life, the protean hysteric passion would be less rife among the middle and higher classes and an immunity granted to many otherwise beautiful girls.... I cannot help indulging in anticipation of the glorious future... We rejoice at the downfall of superstition and the progress of science. The light of learning is not now confined, as in feudal days to "the convent, the cloister and the crown," but is diffused and will go on expanding and brightening 'till the shadows of hysteria...will be entirely dispelled by its flood-like radiance. There is a good day coming.

Good days came soon enough for young Fischer who went on to have a long and successful medical career in Rhode Island where he became a leader in civic and professional affairs.

In July 1838, several years before Messrs. Ayer, Fischer, Tibbets and Page matriculated in Hanover, **Dr. Oliver Wendell Holmes** (see chapter 3) accompanied his friend Ralph Waldo Emerson who'd been invited to give an oration to Dartmouth's literary societies; years later Holmes would recall the "cautious old tenants of the Hanover aviary...[and] the endemic orthodoxy of that place." Nevertheless, OWH was "mightily pleased" to be invited to join Dartmouth's six member medical faculty as professor of anatomy and physiology. He'd recently completed two years studying in Paris and on his return obtained his medical degree from Harvard (1836) and opened a small practice in Boston. When he accepted the Dartmouth position he wrote to a friend, "This is a very excellent appointment and as I do not lecture until next August, I shall have plenty of time to get ready."

Because Oliver Wendell Holmes already had a reputation as a poet, he was invited to give the annual Phi Beta Kappa speech at Dartmouth's next commencement which would occur the week before his first scheduled anatomy lecture. Although his oration was well received, some questioned whether the twenty-nine year old, five foot four inch tall professor wasn't an entering freshman? When Holmes taught in Hanover a professor's salary was $400 for each term, supplemented by ticket sales that students paid directly to their teachers. Anatomists had to provide their own teaching models; at one oral examination, OWW had his students reach into a bag of bones and describe whatever they pulled out - afterwards he gleefully exclaimed, "They can't do that at Harvard." The job required his presence for only fourteen weeks from August through October and when Holmes arrived by stage coach several weeks early he was charmed by the bucolic surroundings: the elm trees, Mt. Ascutney looming in the distance and the village "lying in cataleptic stillness." In later years, he rhapsodized about his "autumnal sojourn by the Connecticut, where it comes loitering down from its mountain fortress like a great Lord."

In Hanover, Professor Holmes met a kindred soul of the same age, the brilliant Elisha Bartlett who also joined the faculty that same year as professor of theory and practice. The two boarded at The Dartmouth Hotel which OWH described as "that caravansary on the bank of the stream where Ledyard launched his log canoe." After delivering forty-four lectures Elisha Bartlett wrote, "the class is respectable and that is about all that can be said" but he was restless and resigned after a single term. Shortly after they'd first met Bartlett described his new friend: "His talk at table is all spontaneous, unpremeditated he pours himself forth...in a perfect torrent. His wit and humour are quite lost in the prodigal exuberance of his thought and language." How much both men valued table talk is suggested in a letter from Bartlett to Holmes (October 1839) that was written several months after Bartlett left Hanover. In it he described his current dining companions: "We had at our *table d'hote* a lot of inane asses, wrongheaded and long eared enough to take away the appetite of a gourmand." For his part, Holmes wrote to Bartlett, "The students looked quite inconsolable and the hotel seemed like a hearse-home."

Later that same year, citing the pressure of his private practice in Boston, and having married two months before the 1840 term began, Holmes also resigned his position. Seven years later he was appointed to chair anatomy and physiology at Harvard Medical School where during the next thirty-five years, he became the school's most popular teacher and one of America's favorite writers and lecturers. No doubt during OWH's two-year sojourn in Hanover, he bubbled over with new ideas that he'd picked up during his stay in Paris (April 1833-October 1835). Legend holds that the school's founder Eleazar Wheelock had entered Hanover's wilderness "to teach the Indian...with a Bible, a drum and five hundred gallons of New England rum," but Professor Holmes brought a stethoscope, a microscope and a skeleton, all purchased in Paris.

His time abroad had been both transformative and delightful. Most young Americans who studied in Paris -- more than 800 during the 1820s through 1850s -- could scarcely understand what their professors were saying but Holmes hired a private language tutor and had a grand time. He wrote to his father about "the Paradise of Paris…I love to talk French, to eat French [and] drink French every now and then." To a friend he confided that he "refreshed himself with making love to a pretty *grisette*." Concerning the French style of medical practice:

> *It was something to have unlearned the pernicious habit of constantly giving poisons to a patient, as if they were good in themselves, of drawing off the blood which he would want in his struggle with disease, of making him sore and wretched with needless blisters, of turning his stomach with unnecessary nauseous draught and mixtures – only because he was sick and something must be done.*

In his inaugural lecture at Dartmouth (August 1, 1839) Professor Holmes, spelled out his medical philosophy that had been formed in Paris. Although this talk is long forgotten, Professor William C. Dowling of Rutgers has described it as a "noteworthy event in American medical history" because the young professor was suggesting that the traditional medical model was outmoded and that received doctrines, dogma and theoretic "systems" were passé. A new era of skeptical empiricism and therapeutic nihilism had dawned in Paris and, according to Dowling, with both Holmes and Bartlett on its faculty "Dartmouth Medical School in 1839 might have claimed with some justice to be the major outpost of Paris medicine in the United States." Perhaps so, but probably only a few of the more alert in the audience that balmy summer day were aware of the import of the lecturer's message while most of their fellow students dozed. Nearly a half century later, in his farewell address to his Harvard students (November 28, 1882), Oliver Wendell Holmes remarked, "Old theories and old men who cling to them, must take themselves out of the way as the new generation with its fresh thoughts and altered habits of mind come forward to take the place of that which is dying out."

While describing some of his early teachers, Holmes singled out Pierre-Charles-Alexandre Louis who during bedside rounds at La Pitié hospital advocated meticulous clinical observation and emphasized data collection on a large number of similar patients – his so-called called "numerical method." OWH wrote home that the French approach was based on three caveats: "not to take authority when I can have facts; not to guess when I can know; not to think a man must take physic because he is sick." Professor Louis taught his students "to love truth, the habit of passionless listening to the teachings of nature, the most careful and searching methods of observation." It was this attitude that young physicians brought back and disseminated to their own students.

Surely the fresh approaches proposed by Holmes and Bartlett must have influenced Dartmouth students. Indeed, Charles Safford's thesis which was written in 1839, the only year that both Holmes and Bartlett lectured in Hanover, employed Pierre Louis's "numerical method" in order to discuss a complicated case. Nevertheless, the four student theses about hysteria described here displayed vestiges of the old way of thinking along with the new and it's not surprising that they retained some of the traditional linkage of hysteria to the uterus or advocated bleeding as an effective remedy, while at the same time acknowledging that new ideas were emerging that were based on scientific evidence.

Although Oliver Wendell Holmes seemed to have had an opinion about almost everything, he never specifically addressed the subject of hysteria. However we can indirectly piece together his attitude from other things he wrote. At the time he was at Dartmouth, OWH was co-editing the American edition of Marshall Hall's *Principles and Practice of Medicine*, Hall being an English physician who wrote extensively about the features of hysteria. Major characters in two of OWH's fictional works displayed typical hysterical features and it was he who coined the expression "as fickle as a female in hysterics." In his Boylston Prize dissertation titled "Neuralgia" (1836) Holmes ridiculed an earlier physician's suggestion that facial neuralgia could be "allied to, or identical to hysteria" because the condition was more common in men than in women, "particularly fishermen and sailors who are anything but hysteric subjects."

In his student days Holmes' mentor Pierre Louis had learned the technique of auscultation directly from René Théophile Hyacinthe Laennec, who'd invented the stethoscope in 1819, and when Holmes returned from Paris, he brought one home as a souvenir. In one of his three Boylston prize essays he described auscultation as "that wonderful art of discovering disease which, as it were, puts a window in the breast through which the vital organs can be seen." But sometimes there could be unexpected complications as OWH described in *The Stethoscope Song – A*

Professional Ballad (1848). This delightful poem describes "a young man in Boston town" recently returned from Paris where he "bought him a stethoscope nice and new, all mounted and finished and polished down, with an ivory cap and a stopper too." Those early models were monaural wooden cylinders and one day "it happened a spider within did crawl and spun him a web of ample size." Later a few "imprudent" flies also took up residence and merry mischief followed as the young doctor mistook the buzzing and rattling he heard as indicating grave illness. Five stanzas within this long ballad, return us to the subject of hysteria – although the condition is not specifically mentioned, the connection is evident:

Then six young damsels, slight and frail,
Received this kind doctor's cares;
They all were getting slim and pale,
And short of breath on mounting stairs.

They all made rhymes with "sighs" and "skies,"
And loathed their puddings and buttered rolls,
And dieted, much to their friends' surprise,
On pickles and pencils and chalk and coals.

So fast their little hearts did bound,
The frightened insects buzzed the more;
So over all their chests he found
The rale sifflant and the rale sonore.

He shook his head. There's a grave disease,--
I greatly fear you all must die;
A slight post-mortem, if you please,
Surviving friends would gratify.

The six young damsels wept aloud,
Which so prevailed on six young men
That each his honest love avowed,
Wherever they all got well again.

Famously skeptical of quacks and frauds of all kinds, OWH seems to have had doubts about the veracity of young damsels, such as the six described above who protested too much and perhaps this also related to his ideas about hysteria as was expressed in a letter to the editor published in the New York Times, June 12, 1881:

> *As for moral and mental manifestations, a hysteric girl will lie so that Sapphira would blush for her, and she could give lessons to a professional pickpocket in the art of stealing. Hysteria may well be described as possession – possession by seven devils, except that this number is quite insufficient to account for all the pranks played by the subjects of this extraordinary malady.*

Dr. Holmes didn't offer any specific suggestion about the fundamental nature of hysteria but, no doubt, he would have approved of on-going research which attempted to correlate anatomic lesions with clinical signs as a way of comprehending the condition. In his inaugural lecture, Holmes explained to his Dartmouth students how far things already had come by 1839 concerning nervous system pathophysiology in general:

> *There was a time when one of the ventricles was considered as the pocket of memory, and the soul was thought to be seated like a charioteer upon a little body of the size of a pea, where it holds the reins of reason in the shape of two little white hands – and grave men believed such things, and knowledge was choked up in volumes that contained long disputes upon such things. Wheresoever sound observation silenced such scholastic babbling, even if it cannot substitute any positive fact in the place of the idle speculations it overturns, it removes a mountain from the path of the student.*

A quarter century after Holmes's criticism of "scholastic babbling" and our four students' dissertations, a so-called "Golden Age of Hysteria" occurred in Paris where the condition achieved near cult status; patients' flamboyant behavior sometimes imitated by chic society women – a la mode. During the 1870s and 1880s the epicenter of this phenomenon was La Salpêtrière, a former gunpowder arsenal which was transformed to a huge storehouse for more than 5,000 miserable women – the demented and deranged mixed with beggars, prostitutes and the dregs of society. The medical director was the imperious neurologist Jean-Martin Charcot who variously described his domain as "this living museum of pathology," "this wilderness of paralysis, spasms and convulsions," "this vast emporium of human suffering."

Charcot had a special interest in the hysterics in his charge and frequently displayed the more interesting cases at weekly medical conferences (*Lecons du Mardi*) that attracted not only physicians but fashionable crowds. Like marionettes they acted out to their puppeteer's command -- barking, posturing, fainting -- and the most theatrical were celebrated like divas. Charcot insisted that these living specimens had an inherited neurologic disorder which predisposed them to classic "stigmata" that he could unmask through hypnosis. Neither madwomen nor malingerers, he believed that they suffered from a real enough disorder, albeit a specific lesion had not yet been identified. At the same time, the famous professor was typical of his misogynist era when women's emotional behavior seemed inexplicable to men – one journalist claimed that a quarter of the women of Paris were hysterics; another called it "the great modern ailment" and many doctors felt they had to protect the weaker sex from their foolish inclinations.

Publishing hundreds of articles on the subject and consulting on thousands of cases, Charcot legitimated hysteria, but when *le maître* died in 1892 his reputation crumbled and his theories were quickly discarded. Twenty years before Charcot, only 1% of La Salpêtrière's inmates were diagnosed with hysteria; during his heyday 17%; twenty years after his death none. That's not to say that the disorder disappeared; it was merely called other things, e.g. conversion reaction, anxiety, panic attack.

Modern medicine no longer talks about hysteria – no respectable physician would use the term – but although Charcot's theories were short-lived within the medical community, not so in the public mind nor in the fertile imaginations of novelists and playwrights. To this very day, novels, plays and movies continue to appear describing characters suffering from the symptoms and signs of hysteria. So it's not surprising that nearing mid-19th century four Dartmouth medical students chose Hysteria for the subject of their dissertations and although they were confused about the nature of the condition, some of their suggestions regarding treatment or prevention were sensible enough – fresh air, exercise, an overseas trip, cheerful company - "early and judicious marriage." In 1847, young Charles Fischer had predicted that a better day was coming: "We rejoice at the downfall of superstition and the progress of science." Nevertheless, despite our more sophisticated, high tech modern approach, an adequate explanation for the enigma of hysteria still is lacking.

9. DOCTEUR DIEU

In June 2015 the Metropolitan Museum of Art in New York mounted a stunning exhibition of ninety paintings and drawings by the famous American artist John Singer Sargent. Dominating one large gallery was a huge portrait titled "Dr. Pozzi at Home" which was painted in 1881. It stood out amidst the generally muted portraits of Sargent's friends and patrons because of its luminous scarlet color - one authority called it an "ode to red." The New York Times' reviewer described, the subject Dr. Samuel-Jean Pozzi as a "glamour-boy gynecologist to the stars." I decided to learn more.

The appearance is not that of a staid physician in black frock coat. It is more that of a self-assured Spanish grandee painted in the style of Velazquez. As one art historian suggested, "This vision of a gorgeous man dressed to match a sumptuous red interior could not be more theatrical. The palate triggers associations of blood, passion, luxury and devilishness while the dressing gown echoes the scarlet robes worn by cardinals."

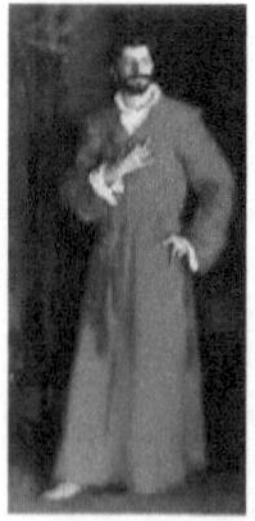

In the full length life-sized portrait (he was more than six feet tall) Dr. Pozzi is a model of masculine virility, resplendent in an ankle length scarlet dressing gown which covers a white night-shirt with ruffled collar and sleeves. An embroidered slipper peaks out from below the robe and the handsome figure is set against a backdrop of crimson drapes. Then 35 years old, the doctor evidently enjoyed posing, while plucking at the robe's collar he looks away from the viewer as if certain that he is having an effect. Aside from Pozzi's bearded face, the viewer's eyes are drawn to his hands - surprisingly slender, almost effeminate - the very same spidery fingers that soon would popularize bimanual pelvic examinations among his medical colleagues (without gloves) which he described as "the most admirable method of investigation that perhaps exists in gynecology." Apparently Pozzi's patients agreed. Because of his good looks, affable charm and cultured demeanor, one female friend called him "the Love Doctor" — his pupils nicknamed him "The Siren" while to his famous lover Sarah Bernhardt he was *Docteur Dieu* (Doctor God.)

Samuel Pozzi may have been a vain dandy in private life, but he was a dedicated and respected physician who during his career published more than 400 journal articles; his 1000 plus pages textbook of gynecology, a standard for more than four decades, was translated into five languages. When only a young doctor, Pozzi wrote to his beloved grandmother that "The study of the sufferings of Man is one of the best, the highest callings that I could have undertaken and my soul is compensated as my heart in accomplishing this mission." He was a disciple of the famed neuroanatomist Paul Broca and although today no familiar eponyms recall Pozzi's name, during his time some considered him to be the "father" of gynecology in France. He established the first surgical service devoted to diseases of women and his ascent up the academic latter culminated in 1901 when he was appointed as the first professor of gynecology at the University of Paris. A medical colleague once described Pozzi as "a powerful and irrepressible force of life whose exuberance nevertheless blended well with a natural grace and courtesy that made him a model for all of who worked with him." He certainly was a splendid sartorial figure on rounds, favoring spotless white overalls and a black surgeon's cap.

Samuel Pozzi was an early advocate of Lister's antiseptic techniques, visited his colleague in Edinburgh to study his techniques first hand and then introduced many of them in Paris with excellent results. In Scotland he not only learned to wash his hands but learned the advantage of using absorbable catgut for suturing and, from then on, he insisted on scrupulous cleanliness in the operating room. Fluent in English, in 1892

Dr. Pozzi made the first of three trips to the United States to learn what new practices were being employed there. He loved the informality and willingness to share of American surgeons, who called him Sam, and he was able to visit the Chicago World's Fair where he sampled such American staples as Aunt Jemima's pancakes, Cracker Jacks and Juicy Fruit chewing gum. Upon his return he introduced many innovations in the about to be rebuilt Broca Hospital: central heating, ventilation of wards, electrification, an aseptic operating room. In these fact-finding excursions he visited the Mayo Clinic, Johns Hopkins and hospitals in St. Louis, Chicago, Boston and Rochester. On Pozzi's last trip in 1909 he visited Alexis Carrel at the Rockefeller Institute in New York City and was intrigued by his expatriate countryman's vascular surgery skill and impressed by Carrel's novel experiments with organ transplantation.

When Sargent and Pozzi first met at a salon in 1880, the artist was 24, the doctor about ten years older. He had recently married a wealthy heiress and the portrait that was commissioned by Pozzi was painted at their luxurious Parisian home which, as was stylish at the time, featured a red interior. Evidently Sargent recognized a kindred aesthete in Pozzi and gave much thought about how to pose him. After its completion the painting was displayed at exhibitions in London and Brussels but reactions were mixed. The hint of eroticism outraged many sober viewers and not all art critics were impressed — one scoffed, "it contains, like a champagne glass filled too quickly, more foam than golden wine." Such reactions didn't disturb Pozzi and although the painting was never publicly displayed in France, it served to enhance the doctor's notoriety as a sensualist. It's tempting to speculate that this didn't inhibit his bedside manner — which one suspects sometimes may have progressed from *beside* to *upon* the beds of wealthy women - however, modern historians insist that Pozzi generally kept his professional and personal services to the ladies separate. As biographer Caroline de Costa concluded, "While Pozzi led a full and active professional life and a full and active social life, the two were clearly demarcated." Another critic Dr. Claude Vanderpooten wrote that "Samuel loved women, loved them passionately, liked everything which is beautiful...blonde or dark, slender or voluptuous...he devoted his life to them."

As a patron of the arts, Samuel Pozzi was a well-known figure in *fin-de-siecle* salons. His friends, acquaintances and patients included Claude Monet, Auguste Rodin, Robert Louis Stevenson, Charles Darwin, Emile

Zola, George Bizet, Marcel Proust, Georges Clemenceau, Alexander Dumas, Alfred Dreyfus, Gustave Eiffel, Anatole France and Marie Curie. The list of his intimates was equally impressive but surely the most famous was Sarah Bernhardt, known to all as "the Divine Sarah." The daughter of a Dutch courtesan and an unknown father, she was the most celebrated actress of her time — perhaps of *any* time — described recently as "the first international superstar."

The two first met at a salon in 1869 when he was a 23 year old medical student while she, two years older, was becoming the toast of Paris. She was flirtatious, seductive and throughout her life would have untold admirers and paramours - marriage never deterred her. But evidently Sarah's great love was *Docteur Dieu* although their torrid, but on again off again affair lasted only for about ten years. Sometimes they would communicate three or four times a day and her feeling was evident in hundreds of letters written by Sarah to Sam (his letters to her were lost) that were described in *The Diva and Doctor God* by Caroline de Costa and Francesca Miller (2010.) What follows here are but a few feverish tidbits:

> *My Sam I love you I love you and I am yours...Come and take me, if it can be done great will be my joy.*

> *My much desired Sam, my beloved master, I am yours to die of love.... I am yours unto madness...*

> *To my Doctor God, to the Being I adore and admire and to whom I would happily give my life...*

But both lovers were ambitious and determined to pursue their respective careers which demanded very different life styles and their passion cooled in 1879 when Pozzi married the wealthy Marie-Therese Loth-Cazalis. This turned out to be a long but unhappy relationship, not helped by his wife's insistence that her meddling mother live with them, nor by Pozzi's frequent absences on medical matters and his absorption with collecting antiquities and coins and pursuing interests in the arts, science, politics and fencing. Although Samuel and Therese retained a civil public relationship and frequently entertained lavishly, in private they battled endlessly and in later years lived apart.

Although the ardor between Sam and Sarah Bernhardt may have lessened after he married Therese (evidently more on his part than hers) the two maintained an active correspondence and he continued to advise the actress on medical matters. In 1898 she refused to permit anyone but Pozzi resect a large ovarian cyst. Sarah also suffered from a chronically infected knee, the result of an injury sustained during a performance, and in 1915 when the pain became unendurable, she wrote this to Samuel:

> *Listen to me, adored friend. I beg you to cut off my leg a little above the knee. Do not protest. I have perhaps ten or fifteen years left. Why condemn me to constant suffering? Why condemn me to inactivity? Even with a celluloid cast I shall be handicapped and won't be able to perform. And horror of horrors, I shall always be in pain.*

Because the 68 year old Dr. Pozzi was away serving in the army, he arranged for an amputation to be performed by a colleague and at about the time of the surgery, Sarah Bernhardt wrote again to her *Docteur Dieu*:

How is it that my infinite love and gratitude over so many years have not actually taken root and blossomed in your heart? How is it that I feel the need to tell you again and again that there is no being dearer to me than you? Can it be, dear friend, that I must open the box of memories we share to let you breathe the perfume of these flowers we gathered together in the garden of Life… I love you with all the vital and intellectual force of my being, and nothing, nothing could change this feeling, greater than Friendship, more divine than Love.

Amputation didn't stop the indomitable diva. She tried several wooden legs but none suited her so she arranged to be carried about by porters on a gilded sedan chair like an empress and went off to entertain the troops going as close to the front as allowed. One admirer reported her being held aloft, "her arms full of roses, her mutilated figure a mass of velvets. She was the personification of undaunted courage." A fellow performer captured the scene this way:

> *The flimsy curtain fluttered open to reveal a wisp of an aging woman propped…in a shabby armchair. Then the wisp began her lines and the miracle took place…Sarah, old, mutilated, once more illuminated a crowd by the rays of her genius…When she wound up her recitation two thousand men rose to their feet cheering…She is greater perhaps in this glowing twilight than in the sparkling days of her apogee.*

Although Samuel Pozzi's charm, intelligence and wit were irresistible to the ladies, his most long-lasting extra-marital affair began during the 1890s when he met Emma Bischoff, a wealthy Jewish socialite. When his wife Therese refused a divorce, she remained the doctor's mistress and travel companion for some twenty-four years until his death in 1918.

At the end of the same gallery in the Metropolitan Museum of Art's exhibition of John Singer Sargent's paintings hung perhaps his most famous portrait, now known as *Madame X.* It caused a sensation when exhibited at the Salon in 1916 - as reported in the *NY Times*, she was "the young Parisian socialite Virginie Amelie Avegno Gautreau, whose 'new woman' image - plunging black dress, lavender-powdered skin, and air of aloof disdain - threatened to send Sargent's reputation off the tracks." Louisiana born of Creole descent, Amelie was reputed to be the most beautiful woman in Paris and was married to a banker twice her age. Because her portrait often has been juxtaposed by museum curators of Sargent exhibits with *Dr. Pozzi at Home*, there were persistent rumors that she was the gynecologist's sometime lover and they certainly were acquaintances. But current historians are adamant that there was never a romantic connection between the two — indeed not all of Samuel Pozzi's soulmates were bedmates and he had many platonic female friends. Sargent's painting of the bare-shouldered voluptuous *Madame* caused such a scandal that the artist fled Paris and resettled in London. Amelie's reputation was ruined and in 1915, shortly after she died in relative obscurity, Sargent sold the portrait to New York's Metropolitan Museum of Art and asked that her name be removed —thus the title *Madame X.*

As an artist John Singer Sargent sometimes was described as a "sensualist" and perhaps this may have carried over to his personal life. He was a confirmed bachelor, painfully shy in public, and it is possible that he was a closeted homosexual. Bernard Berenson suggested that he had a gift for "the sensory revelation of character" and one of Sargent's biographers (T.J. Fairbrother) perceived a "hidden sexuality" and "particular interest in masculinity." But Sargent always insisted that he only painted what he saw, never introducing his own feelings, so we can only imagine the effect that the virile Dr. Pozzi may have had upon him. In later years the two remained friends, corresponding, and the doctor visiting after Sargent's move to London. Sargent's portrait *Dr. Pozzi at Home* remained in the family's possession and was rarely shown in public until it was purchased by Armand Hammer and in 1990 placed on permanent display in Hammer's museum in Los Angeles.

With advancing age, Samuel Pozzi developed a paunch, the black beard transformed to a white goatee and although he still dressed elegantly, no longer as flamboyantly. Then on June 13, 1918, the 72 year old gynecologist was shot to death in his consulting room — not, as one might imagine, by a jealous husband but by a disgruntled patient. About three years earlier Pozzi had removed a scrotal varicocele - a minor procedure, but the man attributed his impotence and other problems to what he perceived to be a failed operation. He insisted that Pozzi correct the problem but the doctor refused because this could not possibly remedy the man's various problems. The enraged lunatic shot his surgeon four times in the abdomen and then killed himself. An emergency laparotomy was unsuccessful and, at Dr. Pozzi's request, he was buried in his military uniform, the Legion of Honor and other medals pinned on his chest — resplendent to the end.

10. MEDICAL MARVEL AND MORAL MONSTER

The following describes a different kind of French Connection than those discussed in the two previous chapters. Adapted from a lecture given in 2015 at The Learning Collaborative, Orangeburg, NY.

On April 14, 1939 the *New York Times* reported that on the previous day New York's Rotary Club gave its Gold Service Award to Dr. Alexis Carrel "in recognition of a life devoted to the amelioration of human suffering." The headline blared that the honoree "*FINDS SOCIETY WAVERING. Future life must be based on Reality.*" Then Dr. Carrel's words were reported in some detail:

> *A new civilization will develop when full use is made through a brain pool of scientific knowledge to replace the present civilization [which] is based on ideologies of the 18th century.... In our civilization we have misfits and feebleminded persons that the people of the 18th century did not take into consideration there are hereditary and physiological traits that make individuals different...If we used scientific insights we might discover a new way of life which would be based on reality. If life is based on reality we cannot fail. If it is based on philosophical or sociological ideologies we will fail as we already have failed. Our present knowledge is too great to be in one mind. It should be coordinated into a brain pool or a sort of composite Aristotle... It is too soon now but it will come because it is absolutely necessary.*

What kind of a person could make such grandiose statements – especially in April 1939? On the very same day as this newspaper account, Franklin Roosevelt wrote a letter to Adolf Hitler requesting the Chancellor to give his personal assurance of peaceful intent so the United States could serve as a "friendly intermediary" and assure thirty-two other nations that they wouldn't be invaded. According to Roosevelt, "Plainly the world is moving toward the moment when this situation must end in catastrophe unless a more rational way of guiding events is found." FDR's request was ridiculed in Berlin and less than five months later Germany invaded Poland. The week before Carrel's talk in New York, Pope Pius XII congratulated Generalissimo Franco for his victory in Spain, Mussolini invaded Albania and Marian Anderson sang before 75,000 people at the Lincoln Memorial. Writing in her daily newspaper column Eleanor Roosevelt's words were muted and almost fatalistic:

> *Here in America, so many miles away, the clouds which hang over other countries are felt and, more and more, the thought seems to come home to us that we are fortunate to live in America. I suppose, however, that no matter where you live or under what conditions, you carry on your daily tasks and adjust yourself to whatever circumstances you may have to meet. Probably this is why human beings survive all kinds of situations. Impossible as it seems today that one could ever survive and adjust to certain things, one will find oneself doing so tomorrow and almost forgetting that other conditions ever prevailed.*

Alexis Carrel's speech to New York's Rotary Club was merely a sampler of his beliefs that had recently been described in the second edition of his international bestseller *Man the Unknown*. Never timid nor humble, in 320 dense pages the surgeon, who had won the Nobel Prize in 1912 for his work on vascular suturing and transplantation of blood vessels and organs, told how to improve the human race through psychology, nutrition, exercise, education and spiritual enrichment. When the book's first edition appeared in October 1935, it was second in sales only to *Gone With The Wind* and the author's face appeared on the cover of *Time Magazine*. The outspoken Dr. Carrel was well aware of world events and in the preface of the second edition his words were prophetic and apocalyptic:

The book is having the paradoxical destiny of becoming more timely while it grows older. Its significance has increased continually. The real significance of the events taking place in Europe and in this country is not yet understood by the public...The crisis is due neither to the presence of Mr. Roosevelt in the White House nor to that of Hitler in Germany nor of Mussolini in Rome. It comes from the very structure of civilization. It is a crisis of man. Man is not able to manage the world derived from the caprice of his intelligence. He has no other alternative than to remake this world according to the laws of life. He must adopt his environment to the nature of his organic and mental activities and renovate his habits of existence. To progress again, man must remake himself...Otherwise, modern society will join ancient Greece and the Roman Empire in nothingness. And the basis of this renovation can be found only in the knowledge of our body and soul...He cannot remake himself without suffering. For he is both the marble and the sculptor. In order to uncover his true visage, he must shatter his own substance with heavy blows of his hammer.

(The following statements from Carrel's book are out of order and slightly edited.)

The human race is degenerating morally and mentally, indifferent to everything but money. The only possible remedy is a much more profound knowledge of ourselves...But there's reason for hope because, after all, the ancestral potentialities still exist in the germ plasm of their weak offspring.

Men are not born equal... A great race must propagate its best elements to form a better human stock. Many inferior individuals have been conserved through the efforts of hygiene and medicine and the only way to obviate the disastrous predominance of the weak is to develop the strong.

The feeble-minded and the man of genius should not be equal before the law. The stupid, the unintelligent...those incapable of attention, of effort, have no right to a higher education.

Eugenics is indispensable for the perpetuation of the strong. It asks for the sacrifice of many individuals...Philosophical and sentimental prejudices must give way before necessity.

The free practice of eugenics could lead not only to the development of stronger individuals but also strains endowed with more endurance, intelligence and courage. These strains should constitute an aristocracy from which great men probably would appear.

What's needed is a high council living in seclusion like monks... audacious men of science, unafraid of resorting to extreme, even ruthless measures. They should be free from research or teaching responsibilities and dedicate their lives to contemplation of our habits and thoughts...Our destiny is in our hands. Humanity's attention must turn from the machines of the world of inanimate matter to the body and the soul of man...On the new road, we must now go forward.

Alexis Carrel noted that upon this "new road" the defenders of the body and soul of a great race should be descendants of bold men – the likes of crusaders, revolutionaries, great criminals, financial and industrial magnates. Those deemed worthy should have their lives extended while the dregs of society would be "*humanely and economically disposed of in small euthanistic institutions supplied with the proper gasses...Why preserve useless and harmful beings?*" In fairness, by "harmful" Carrel meant those guilty of criminal acts who were refractory to such corporal punishment as "lashing." However, the term "useless" was a code word frequently employed in those days by eugenicists and later by Nazis to characterize the unwanted other, the "unfit," the mentally ill, epileptics, homosexuals, gypsies, Jews. And although Carrel was referring to individual executions by using "proper gasses", it should be noted that in this country, between the 1920s and 2010, hundreds of criminals were executed in gas chambers and it remains a legal option in several states. Nevertheless, Carrel wasn't thinking exclusively about eliminating criminals; at various other times he said the following:

-Civilization is already encumbered with those who should be dead: the weak, the diseased and the fools.

> *-Natural selection no longer plays its part because the weak are saved as well as the strong.*
> *-Perhaps it would be effective to kill off the worst and keep the best, as we do in breeding dogs.*
> *-The old order must die so that the new order lives.*
> *-The fight of man against death will perhaps succeed too well. For the artificial postponement of death of a large number of individuals would be a far greater calamity than death itself*

Alexis Carrel believed that prolonged life should be reserved for the select few, the "builders of civilizations," and he had no doubt that there would be many worthy candidates for this new ruling caste: "Even in our own base and egotistical age, thousands of men and women still follow, on the battlefield, in the monastery or in that abomination of desolation the modern city, the path of heroism and holiness." He hoped to establish an "Institute of Man", a think tank staffed by a "high council" of experts who not only would study mankind but *mold* it. All Americans under age 30 would be evaluated to determine who should or should not be permitted to propagate – only the best strains allowed to do so. During the 1930s when Carrel praised Nazi Germany for its "energetic measures" to prevent contamination of the human race, his was not a lone voice; indeed his views were shared by many Americans, thousands flocked to his lectures and millions read his book. Was Alexis Carrel a moral monster? a fascist? a Nazi? an anti-Semite? a mad scientist? -- or merely a misguided elitist? Because seventy-five years later, it's difficult to say with clarity, let's consider his story in greater detail.

Alexis Carrel was born June 28, 1873 to a prosperous and devout Catholic family near Lyon (Lyons) the great silk production center. When he was a twenty year old medical student in Lyon, an anarchist stabbed the president of France, Sadi Carnot, severing his portal vein and he bled to death. Young Carrel realized that the surgical techniques of the time were insufficient and took lessons from an expert embroiderer who taught him to use tiny needles and fine thread. He practiced diligently and developed a delicate suturing technique which permitted anastomosing blood vessels as small as a millimeter in diameter and in 1902, when only an assistant in the anatomy department, he read a paper before the local medical society describing his method which when widely applied later would revolutionize microvascular surgery.

In 1903 the young doctor was invited to ride "the sick train" which took thousands of pilgrims to the famous Lourdes shrine. He was puzzled by hundreds of miracle cures that had been reported during the 19th century and while on the train personally observed the swollen abdomen of a teenage girl, presumably near death from tuberculous peritonitis, shrink down within a half hour after the nuns sprinkled holy water on her belly. Dr. Carrel couldn't believe his eyes and published what he'd witnessed, concluding that there were phenomena in medicine that could not be explained by science alone. The clergy attacked him for being skeptical while the medical establishment called him gullible and blackballed him for academic promotion. Nevertheless, throughout his life Carrel remained fascinated with miracle cures and frequently revisited Lourdes.

Fed up with the politics of clinical medicine in France, he pursued other interests and in 1904 left for Canada where he briefly considered becoming a rancher. However, he soon had second thoughts, worked briefly in Chicago, and in September 1905 accepted an invitation from Dr. Simon Flexner, medical director of the brand new Rockefeller Institute for Medical Research, to join him in New York where he would work for the next thirty-three years. Early on his animal experiments were criticized by anti-vivisectionists but their objections were somewhat quelled in 1909 after he performed a daring bedside anastomosis of the popliteal vein of a dying three day old infant directly to the radial artery of her physician father. Both survived the desperate transfusion which was performed in the doctor's West Side apartment and for many critics this remarkable feat established that animal research could have practical human benefits.

At Rockefeller, Carrel continued doing various organ transplants and in 1910 performed the first coronary bypass operation on a dog. Although animal surgery was technically quite easy for him, most animals rejected the transplants and died and Carrel realized that something was happening at the cellular level. This prompted his subsequent research on tissue culture and in 1912, when he won the Nobel Prize for Medicine and Physiology, at age 39 he was the youngest individual to receive that honor and the first physician working in the United States. The Nobel committee noted that his work provided the "means of curing the wounds and maladies that so harm the human species." In his Nobel Lecture Carrel acknowledged the contributions of predecessors and continuing problems related to tissue culture which hindered practical application. However, he predicted that these would be surmounted and "render possible the benefits to humankind which we hope to see accomplished in the future."

While visiting France at the onset of World War I Carrel was called to active duty. He was disturbed by seeing men dying from contaminated wounds and overcame French bureaucracy to start a small research hospital that was partially funded by the Rockefeller Foundation. He collaborated with the English chemist Henry Dakin who had developed a hypochlorite irrigating solution which when used along with surgical debridement and scrupulous asepsis transformed the management of war wounds. As at other times during his long career, Carrel was criticized for taking more credit than was his and not acknowledging the important contributions of others – in this case Henry Dakin.

After the War and back at the Rockefeller Institute, he operated in a labyrinth of rooms on the building's top floor that were brightly lit by skylights. In order to combat the sun's glare, he painted walls, floors and equipment black and all workers wore black masks and hooded robes and the dramatic effect must have been sinister. Carrel had a life-long talent for offending people. He was brusque, aloof and had a genius for self-promotion which was resented by his peers. His most widely publicized experiment involved cells from an embryonic chicken heart that was kept alive in vitro, for 34 years, finally discarded two years after Carrel's death. The press had a field day speculating about the "immortal" chicken heart and what it might portend for humans. Every year one newspaper would run a Happy Birthday column to the chicken heart and an obituary when it "died."

In November 1930, Charles Lindbergh came to visit Dr. Carrel at the Institute. As was his eccentric custom, at their first meeting Carrel silently scrutinized the much younger man's face for several minutes before he passed muster. It was about three years since Lindbergh's epic trans-Atlantic flight but now he had a personal agenda far removed from aviation. His sister-in-law had a dysfunctional heart valve as a result of rheumatic heart disease and Lindbergh hoped that Carrel could suggest a way of repairing the valve surgically, like could be done with engine valves. When told that such a procedure was impossible without the aid of an artificial heart, the mechanically gifted Lindbergh proposed to build one. A patient's heart would have to be removed, repaired outside the body and then replaced and he envisioned a pulsatile pump that could sustain life during surgery. At the same time, Carrel invited Lindbergh to collaborate in other research already under way, searching for methods to keep "alive" and functioning excised portions of animal tissues and even entire organs.

For Lindbergh, the much older Carrel was a father figure; for Carrel here was the son he never had. They were an odd couple in physical appearance – the tall, thin flyer and the elfin, bald Frenchman who wore a black beret and pince-nez glasses. But in some ways they were a perfect match. Both thought of the body as a living machine that was made of replaceable parts and although it took Lindbergh four years to perfect his "Life Chamber" apparatus, when he did, they were able to keep various organs "alive" for days or weeks at a time. In September 1935 when Dr. Carrel's face appeared on the cover of *Time Magazine* the accompanying article described the semi-secret collaboration of these two celebrities. In June 1938, the colleagues, described as "Men in Black," appeared together on *Time Magazine's* cover with their hand-blown glass heart pump between them -- and the next year the pump was displayed at New York World's Fair.

Alexis Carrel's book *Man The Unknown* was translated into nineteen languages and appeared in a condensed series in the *Readers Digest*. In it he acknowledged that although his interest in clairvoyance, telepathy and the power of prayer were unorthodox. Although "scientists will consider my interest to be puerile or insane" he didn't hesitate discussing his ideas because these phenomena are "real." Predictably, after reading a book review in the *New York Times* a prominent psychiatrist wrote a letter to the editor objecting to Carrel's remark that prayer can cure cancer and other ailments within a few minutes.

As early as 1911, when testifying at a meeting of the American Breeders Association, Alexis Carrel said, "The diseases of the mind are a serious menace...They are to be feared, not only because they increase the number of criminals, but chiefly because they profoundly weaken the dominant white races." The ideal solution would be the suppression of each of these individuals "as soon as he has proven himself to be dangerous." He endorsed a program of "voluntary" eugenics; i.e. discouraging the "unfit" from marrying. As a social Darwinist he advocated weeding out the unfit while encouraging the elite to multiply: "a great race must propagate its best elements." Eugenicists like him believed in better breeding practices; according to him, "Eugenics is indispensable for the perpetuation of the strong." Once Carrel wrote, "The herd always profits by the ideas and inventions of the elite. Instead of leveling organic and mental inequalities, we should…construct greater men. Although he advocated "positive" eugenics and, in individual cases sometimes even "negative" eugenics, he never sanctioned mass involuntary sterilization or euthanasia of sick or defective children or adults as already was being done in Nazi Germany during the 1930s.

When Carrel's chief supporter Simon Flexner retired in October 1935, he was replaced as director of the Rockefeller Institute by Herbert Gasser. The new director was appalled by Carrel's extramural activities, particularly the speech he gave about "The Mystery of Death" to an overflow crowd at the New York Academy of Medicine (December 12, 1935) with several thousand people unable to get inside. The next day the *Times* breathlessly reported on page one that Carrel had predicted that although death was not conquerable it could be postponed for years – indeed by placing a human in a state of suspended animation, "a period of centuries may become one of the realities of tomorrow." He speculated that in the future if an old man was given the glands of a still-born infant or the blood of a young man, he might be rejuvenated. Moreover, he criticized medically assisted prolongation of life for burdening civilized countries with those "who should be dead" – early death described as a builder of civilization since it eliminated "the weak, the diseased and the fools."

One week after Dr. Carrel's lecture at the Academy of Medicine, the liberal journalist Walter Lippman spoke in the same auditorium on "Aspects of a Philosophy of Government in a Sick World." Current events in Europe certainly were on his mind and although he didn't Alexis Carrel by name, surely he was aware of the previous week's event. After explaining that governments should avoid social engineering and that humility is the beginning of wisdom, Lippman's concluding remarks were pointed:

> *Without [recognizing their limits] men will use political power for ends that government cannot realize, and in the vanity of their delusions fall into the manner of cruelty, disorder, and waste. They will have forgotten to respect the nature of living things, and in their ambition to be gods among men they will affront the living god. They will not have learned that those who would be more than human end by being less than human.*

Herbert Gasser was not alone in objecting to the publicity-prone Dr. Carrel who not only trumpeted his own work but discussed politics and education and spoke positively about spiritualists and clairvoyants. Most of the Rockefeller Institute's research scientists shunned the limelight and were taken aback by their outspoken colleague, but Alexis Carrel also had supporters at the Institute. Among them was a young German immigrant Richard Bing, who as a youth had been inspired by reading *Arrowsmith* to take up experimental cardiology. In 1935, while doing investigative studies in Copenhagen, Dr. Bing was invited by Carrel to join him and Lindbergh on their pump studies in New York. (Bing was half-Jewish and this afforded him an opportunity to escape Nazi Germany.) Writing some five decades later, the by-now eminent Dr. Bing recalled Carrel as "a kind, understanding and humane person," a generous mentor who taught him tissue culture techniques which he employed in his own illustrious career. He recalled that his boss admired forceful autocratic personalities [not including FDR] and once remarked that he'd like to become a dictator in some South American nation.

Richard Bing remarked that "things were not easy for Carrel at the Rockefeller Institute which might have been for reasons of his own doing… [because] he was a scientist who believed in nonscientific things." He was a strong believer in the power of mind over body and once made Bing and others sit around a heavy table and attempt to lift it with one hand. They couldn't but then he asked them to count to ten while concentrating on the task and they lifted the table easily. Dr. Bing concluded, "There were certainly few other scientists of an equally contrasting, scintillating and controversial personality. Providence has provided that his scientific work endures, while his controversial personal features have faded into the background."

In 1939 Dr. Gasser invoked a mandatory retirement age of sixty-five which, although it effected others beside Carrel, he took personally. He complained in a letter to an influential friend about "Jewish influences" – after all Gasser was half Jewish. This was denied after an investigation by the Rockefeller Foundation's lawyers but certainly Gasser was relieved to eliminate the Frenchman's expensive animal research laboratory which included a vast "mousery" that housed some 12,000 rodents fed special diets to test their resistance to cancer and other diseases and bred for physical strength.

In fact, during the 1930s the Rockefeller Institute had a liberal policy toward employing senior Jewish scientists at a time when American medical schools generally did not. About one third of the Institute's twenty-two member research staff had Jewish origins although, almost to a man, they were assimilated, non-observant and unsympathetic with Zionists who were perceived as being warmongers. – the likes of Phoebus Levine, Alexander Wiener, Jacques Loeb, Alfred Cohn, Samuel Meltzer and Michael Heidelberger. Also among them was Karl Landsteiner who after emigrating from Austria in 1922, worked at the Institute and in 1940 was awarded the Nobel Prize for his discovery of human blood groups. When Landsteiner was a youngster his family had converted to Catholicism and in 1937 when he was included in a *Who's Who in American Jewry*, he threatened a lawsuit of $100,000 on the grounds that his teenage son might be shocked to discover his Jewish ancestry and subjected to humiliation.

Both the Jewish director Simon Flexner and his equally famous brother Abraham were avid eugenicists and, although they never denied their roots, they were more concerned with fitting in with the WASP elite than with the fortunes of their kinsmen. Simon strongly supported Carrel's work and used the favorable publicity given to his trophy Nobel Laureate to promote the Institute and impress the Rockefeller patrons to keep their money flowing. For his part, after being involuntarily retired from the Rockefeller Foundation's Graduate Education Board in 1928, Abraham Flexner went on to found the Institute for Advanced Study in Princeton and appointed Alexis Carrel to his Board of Directors as a guaranteed yes-man.

According to one of Charles Lindbergh's biographers, he once wrote,

> *Whenever the Jewish percentage of the total population becomes too high, a reaction seems to invariably occur. It is too bad because a few Jews of the right type are, I believe, an asset to any country...If an anti-Semitic movement starts in the United States, it may go far* [not too far]. *It will certainly affect the good Jews along with the others.*

Alexis Carrel would have agreed with Lindbergh that a few Jews of "the right type" could be an asset – men like his friend Emanuel Libman, the famous cardiologist at Mount Sinai Hospital. In 1932, at a testimonial dinner on the occasion of Libman's sixtieth birthday, Carrel was unable to attend but sent a laudatory message in which he spoke admiringly about Old Testament prophets as "strong lone figures." Including Libman among contemporary Jewish luminaries such as Einstein and Cardozo, he concluded simply that, "Libman is medicine itself." In a letter to the activist rabbi Stephen S. Wise, who had praised his book as "epochal' and an "oasis of beauty," Carrel noted that "We Christians will always respect the Jews who are proud of being Jews, who recognize that they differ profoundly from us, that they are a people, and a great people."

Every summer Dr. Carrel and his wife vacationed on Saint-Gildas, a 100 acre island off the barren Brittany coast which they'd purchased with money from his Nobel Prize. Exhausted by suffocating publicity after the kidnapping and murder of their infant son in 1932 and the subsequent manhunt and trial of Bruno Hauptmann, the Lindberghs went into self-imposed exile in England and in 1938 purchased Illeic, a 40 acre islet adjacent to Saint-Gildas. As if in a stark Ingmar Bergmann movie, the two friends sometimes would sit alone on their private islands, staring out through mist and surf and meditating about the "crisis" of civilization. Lindbergh could walk several hundred yards across the isthmus separating their enclaves or if the tide was high would row across. Perhaps they may perceived of themselves as Nietzschian *ubermenshen* but even supermen sometime crave solitude or a safe haven from prying eyes and *paparazzi.*

Charles Lindbergh was particularly taken with Carrel's ideas about the superiority of the white race. In turn, Carrel viewed Lindbergh as a "savant" who proved his theory that those capable of greatness in one area could be equally great in other endeavors. Their goal was to graduate from rodents to primates to humans in their experiments at prolonging life and in 1938 they considered visiting the mental institution in Vineland, New Jersey in order to "look over the prospects." However, by 1939 the two men's paths were about to diverge. In his five visits to Germany during the 1930s Lindbergh was impressed by the discipline and precision of the new order. He was wined, dined and courted by the high command and became convinced that no one could defeat the Luftwaffe. Usually when they met, Carrel did most of the talking, but back in Brittany after his most recent inspection trip to Europe, Lindbergh was impatient discussing biological research and race betterment through diet and controlled reproduction. Now he was obsessed with the looming political crisis and eager to advise western political and military leaders – Franklin Roosevelt, Neville Chamberlain, Joseph Kennedy, et al -- of the futility of challenging the Nazi war machine. He believed that Hitler was a "great man," albeit a fanatic, and that it was better to avoid confrontation and acquiesce to the Fuhrer's demands. As Lindbergh saw it, a major problem in America was that Jewish propaganda in Jewish owned newspapers was exaggerating the negatives. On the other hand, Carrel felt that non-intervention was foolish and said that Lindbergh was naïve and "committing suicide with the stupidities he is uttering."

With the onset of war in Europe, Lindbergh became the leading spokesman of the isolationist America First movement. Imbued with Alexis Carrel's eugenic ideas, he felt that war did have one virtue -- it was a way of weeding out the weak. But Carrel retained his French hatred of Les *Bosch* and well remembered the brutality of war from his experiences during World War I. But the two friends agreed that the Soviets posed an even greater threat to civilization than the Germans and that western Jews were war mongering because most of them were communists.

Alexis Carrel's last six years were shrouded in controversy. In 1942 he opened in Paris The French Foundation for Study of Human Problems – usually referred to as The Carrel Foundation – which was funded by the Vichy government. Presumably, the institute's mission was to improve the lot of French children but it also would serve as a laboratory to test his eugenicist ideas – after all, war may have been bestial but it did provide an opportunity to promote the strongest and best. Some latter day apologists, claimed that it was necessary for Carrel to cooperate with the Petain government in order to permit his research institute to function and that he wasn't sympathetic with the excesses of Nazi behavior.

In August 1944 the new French Minister of Health, in an effort to "purify" his department of former collaborators, dismissed the 71 year old Dr. Carrel from his position as head of the Foundation for Study of Human Relations. As he was quoted in the New York Times (Aug 31, 1944): "I was living tranquilly in the United States when I decided that France needed me. I came and founded my institutes for the children of my country and put my theories into practice…I had one aim and I reached it. I am convinced I did not do anything against France." In 1944, broken and depressed, he died of heart failure at age 71 and his body was transported to his island home on the Brittany coast. Historians have been divided about Carrel's final years – some hailed him as a patriot, others called him a scoundrel. Regardless, his name soon was forgotten by most people.

Several of Alexis Carrel's books (which were published posthumously by his wife) became fodder for right-wing conservatives, racists and unreformed eugenicists. During the 1980s his ideas were politicized in France when the xenophobic Jean-Marie LePen praised him as the "first modern ecologist" and described his own followers as "the heirs of Alexis Carrel." In response the head of the University of Lyon's medical school, which in 1969 had been named after Alexis Carrel, declared that his philosophy was unworthy of the Hippocratic tradition: "If we fail to see Carrel's 'barbaric project' for what it was, medicine would be deprived of its civilizing mission and become an instrument of a totalitarian big brother." Subsequently, the school's name was changed to honor Rene Laennec, the inventor of the stethoscope.

After their last meeting in January 1941, Lindbergh and Carrel went their separate ways. Shortly after the war's end, Lindbergh visited Saint-Gildas where Mme. Carrel showed him his friend's humble grave. And nearly three decades later in 1973, when Charles Lindbergh, now 71 years old, spoke at the Alexis Carrel Centennial Conference in Washington, he recalled:

> *I came to ask his advice about problems I had encountered in designing an artificial heart for use during operations...I soon found Carrel himself even more fascinating than the laboratory projects I pursued in his department of experimental surgery. There seemed to be no limit to the breadth and penetration of his thought.... According to his mood, Carrel could work with a precision that caused the admiration of the scientific world, or he could speak with an abandon that brought criticism heaping on his shoulders. He might straighten his back and assert that 'all surgeons are butchers,' and that 'all people are fools,' or sit at his desk and write that 'on the scale of magnitudes man is placed midway between the atom and the star.'...In eulogizing Carrel, one might emphasize his skill as a surgeon, his pioneering work in the fields of tissue and organ culture, his treatment of the wounded in World War I, his suturing of blood vessels which brought him the Nobel Prize, his perception and his depth of vision. Personally, I can say that he had the most stimulating mind I have ever met.*

About a year later Charles Lindbergh died of lymphoma. When his doctors at Columbia could do nothing more, he overruled their orders and had himself flown to his estate on Maui where he orchestrated his final days. Like his mentor, he was buried modestly in his island paradise far from the "civilized" world. Perhaps the most balanced assessment of Alexis Carrel appeared in a book review written in 1997 by the famed heart surgeon Denton A. Cooley:

Rightly deemed a scientific genius, he was also part showman savant, mystic and ascetic. Despite his genuine religious bent and his preoccupation with life's ultimate questions, his behavior lacked many of the qualities associated with true greatness of soul. Moreover his elitist social philosophy was narrow and potentially chilling. As a medical scientist and researcher, however, Carrel has had few equals. Here his greatness is undisputed and modern medicine and its beneficiaries owe him an immense debt.

11. A CAUTIONARY TALE: THE EUGENICS MOVEMENT IN NEW JERSEY

Adapted from remarks made at a symposium held in New Brunswick in 2015.

As originally conceived by Francis Galton, eugenics (meaning well born) evolved from evolutionary biology with the goal of improving the human gene pool; in effect, scientific cultivation of superior beings. However, this idealistic agenda became perverted as emphasis shifted from encouraging the well-bred to multiply to preventing society's less fortunate from propagating at all. Early in the 20th century most Americans accepted as fact that mental illness, crime and poverty were inherited but could be cured by manipulating reproduction. Eugenics dominated intellectual discourse and these ideas were widely held and taught in universities. Some social scientists and religious leaders spoke in apocalyptic terms as if the fate of civilization was at stake – it was necessary to preserve the "racial stock."

During the late 19th century, mental defectives (including epileptics) were segregated on large tracts of land and housed in small decentralized cottages. Two of the biggest of these "colonies" or "villages" were located in New Jersey at The Vineland School for Feebleminded Girls and Boys (founded in 1887) and the State Village for Epileptics at Skillman (1898) where leaders collaborated with the Eugenics Records Office at Cold Springs Harbor, L.I. to study the "pedigrees" of their charges. Indeed, New Jersey was more than a microcosm of what was happening elsewhere - the state played a central role in disseminating information about the importance of eugenics in order to "save the American way of life."

NEW JERSEY TIMELINE

1906: Henry Goddard, appointed to head research at Vineland, modifies Alfred Binet's IQ test and uses it to classify "morons" (a term he coined) who function at an 8 to 12 year old level, "idiots" who function at a 2 year old level and "imbeciles," midway between the others. He reports that two thirds of the feebleminded have inherited their defect and after testing immigrants at Ellis Island, writes "We are getting the poorest of each race." Goddard's later article *The Jackson Whites. A Study in Racial Degeneracy* (1911) describes the "loose ways" of an inbred mix of Indians, former slaves, prostitutes and vagabonds living in Bergen County's Ramapo Mountains.

1911: Leaders at Skillman and Vineland lobby for "An act to authorize and provide for the sterilization of idiots, imbeciles morons, epileptics, rapists and certain criminals and "other defectives." New Jersey's legislature approves and on April 21, 1911 Gov. Woodrow Wilson, who wishes to suppress "citizens of the wrong type, signs the bill into law, the fourth state to do so. The law requires the governor to appoint a three member "Board of Examiners" at each institution which would meet periodically to determine for whom "procreation is inadvisable."

1912: Henry Goddard publishes a book that focuses on the pedigree of a mythical "Kallikak" family living in the Pine Barrens. Later Elizabeth Kite, one of Goddard's field workers, publishes a report based on two years of visits she'd made to cabins in the Pine Barrens and describes the locals as "lazy, lustful and cunning." When New Jersey's Governor Felder visits the area, he is shocked by the number of inbred "Pineys" who lead "lawless and scandalous lives, till they have become a race of imbeciles, criminals and defectives." He proposes to the legislature that the Pine Barrens be segregated from the rest of New Jersey because it produces so many persons who inevitably become public charges.

1912: Bleecker Van Wagenen, a trustee of the Vineland School, chairs the Committee on Sterilization of the American Breeders Association whose goal is to "purge the blood of the American people." Speaking in London at the First International Eugenics Congress, his report "The Best Practical Means for Cutting Off the Defective Germ-Plasm in the Human Population" declares that people of "defective inheritance should be eliminated from the human stock." It asserts that three million Americans of "inferior blood" are not yet in institutions and seven million more – 10% of the total population – carry hereditary maladies; all are "totally unfitted to become parents of useful citizens." Van Wagenen supports killing undesirables but concedes that state sterilization laws will face constitutional challenges, that some research has been premature or flawed and more work needs to be done.

1912: In Zurich, Edward Johnstone (Superintendent of Vineland) boasts that public opinion in New Jersey has swung strongly in favor of the eugenicist approach: "This is the spirit of the legislature of New Jersey and the people of New Jersey. I believe today...we know more about the problem of the feeble-minded than any state in the Union."

1912: The NJ Committee on Provision for the Feeble-minded & Epileptics reports that feeble-minded women average twice as many children as normals....60-90% of cases of feeblemindedness is hereditary and is associated with alcoholism, tuberculosis, syphilis, prostitution and law-breaking of every kind - 7.5% of repeat juvenile offenders are epileptics "in whom the sexual instinct develops abnormally early and in a pronounced manner."

1913: David Weeks, Skillman's medical director, plans to perform a salpingectomy on Alice Smith, a young epileptic resident, but the case Is appealed (*Smith v. Board of Examiners*). New Jersey Supreme Court Justice Charles Garrison (a former MD) finds the statute to be immoral, unconstitutional, "palpably inhumane" and might be abused, but the court's decision applies only to epileptics residing in state-run institutions. Eugenicists threaten to appeal to the U.S. Supreme Court but don't so New Jersey is the first state to overturn its sterilization law and no one was ever sterilized in the state against their will. Nevertheless, the eugenics movement remains very much alive.

1914: New Jersey's "Committee on Provision for the Feeble-Minded and Epileptic" is recast as a national committee based at Vineland. Its director Joseph Byers declares "Never before in any state [as NJ] has there been such wide-spread interest in, and knowledge of, the feebleminded." Vineland's Alexander Johnson is appointed field secretary and over the next three years crisscrosses the country warning "anyone who would listen" about the menace posed by the feebleminded. Nearly 20,000 people hear his message in more than 100 lectures given in New Jersey alone; nationwide, he gives more than 1,100 lectures. Johnson later recalled, "The task was to force upon the attention of the whole people the facts we knew; to convince them of the validity of our methods and of the duty of every state to its feeble minded; and to induce each to discharge that duty fully."

1919: Henry Goddard gives four public lectures on "Human Efficiency and Levels of Intelligence" at Princeton University. Using data from the U.S. Army's IQ tests from WWI, he disputes the Bolshevik "Red Menace": "Socialism is a beautiful theory but the facts must be faced…Intelligence, class and wealth do count; the best should lead. Equal distribution of wealth is absurd because differences in intelligence both explain and justify material differences."

1921: Princeton biologist Edwin G. Conklin writes that in this era of rampant immigration, "God may have withdrawn His ancient promise to His radiant American bride, His new Israel, since she failed to keep herself pure…If God had only continued to sift the nations for our benefit, or if our fathers had exercised only reasonable caution…We might have had here only the choicest blood and the highest types of culture of all lands, we might have replaced the slow and wasteful methods of natural selection by intelligent selection and thus have enormously advanced and hastened human evolution…That chance has gone forever."

1923: Princeton psychology professor Carl Brigham writes in *A Study of American Intelligence*: "In a very definite way, the results which we obtain by interpreting the Army data by means of the race hypothesis support Mr. Madison Grant's thesis of the superiority of the Nordic type… Our figures would rather tend to disprove the popular belief that the Jew is highly intelligent." (Five years later Brigham refuted his own data and rejected eugenics, but by then the damage was done — Congress had passed restrictive immigrations laws largely based on his work.)

1932: George Kennan (Princeton): "Nothing good can come out of modern civilization, in the broad sense. We have only a group of more or less inferior races, incapable of coping adequately with the environment which technical progress has created…No amount of education and discipline can effectively improve conditions as long as we allow the unfit to breed copiously and to preserve their young."

1937: Marian S. Olden of Princeton, an outspoken birth control advocate, founds the Sterilization League of New Jersey. She argues that misguided policies have interfered with natural selection and aided survival of "human weeds": "Defectives are menacing our better stock." Olden claims that the USA has become the "dumping ground" for Europe's "subnormal" population who are prone to crime, mental illness and are promiscuous. She admires Nazi programs and several times introduces compulsory sterilization bills which are rejected, largely due to Catholic opposition.

1981: In the case of Lee Ann Grady, a 19 year old with Down's Syndrome whose parents want her sterilized, New Jersey's Supreme Court rules unanimously that courts, not parents, must decide whether the sterilization of mentally incompetent persons is in the subject's best interest and whether the affected person was incapable of participating in the decision.

2006: Peter Singer, professor of bioethics at Princeton, whose utilitarian philosophy argued for euthanizing infants who have "serious disability," describes "the mixed blessing of genetic choice." Concerning genetic engineering:

> *Many will condemn this as a resurgence of "eugenics", the view, especially popular in the early 20th century, that hereditary traits should be improved through active intervention. So it is, in a way, and in the hands of authoritarian regimes, genetic selection could resemble the evils of earlier forms of eugenics, with their advocacy of odious, pseudoscientific official policies, particularly concerning "racial hygiene.*
>
> *In liberal, market driven societies, however, eugenics will not be coercively imposed by the state for the collective good. Instead, it will be the outcome of parental choice and the workings of the free market. The most alarming implication of this mode of genetic selection, however, is that only the rich will be able to afford it. The gap between rich and poor, already a challenge to our ideas of social justice, will become a chasm that mere equality of opportunity will be powerless to bridge. That is not a future that any of us should approve.*

EUGENICS BEYOND NEW JERSEY

1869: Francis Galton (Charles Darwin's cousin) asserts that the same principles of breeding show dogs and race horses can be applied "to produce a highly gifted race of men by judicious marriages during several consecutive generations." He believes that intelligence, talent and character all are inherited, that "it is a duty we owe to humanity to investigate the range of that power and to exercise it in a way that, without being unwise toward ourselves, shall be most advantageous to future inhabitants of the earth."

1871: Charles Darwin laments the wide spread use of small pox vaccination because it ensures the survival of the weak which is "highly injurious to the race of man…. Except for man himself, hardly anyone is so ignorant as to allow the worst animals to breed." Darwin adapts philosopher Herbert Spencer's term "survival of the fittest." If human society is to become fit, than the logical humane thing is to get rid of the unfit.

1877: Richard Dugdale's book *The Jukes*, a study of a rural New York State family, supports a popular view that disease, pauperism and immorality are inherited traits.

1883: Galton coins the term "eugenics" (well born) for the science of "improving the stock." He suggests it as "the religion of the future…a secular faith" and declares that medical care and misguided social policies have "interrupted the natural struggle for existence by artificially preserving the weak and defective." Europeans are superior to "the lower races" – Jews are described as "parasites," negroes as "childish simpletons."

1900: Gregor Mendel's work with heredity is rediscovered some 40 years after it was performed. By cross-pollinating pea plants Mendel had established the Law of Dominance from which the word "genetics" is coined.

1903: The American Breeders Association (funded by Harriman and Rockefeller money) promotes the value to society of "superior" blood and the menace of "inferior" blood. They say the feebleminded account for most crime and immorality in our civilization.

1903: Theodore Roosevelt: Anglo-Saxons are committing "race suicide" by not replenishing their stock in adequate numbers: "The Jew, the Russian, the Hungarian [and] the Italian are darkly outshading the Americanized descendants of the English…the Germans and the Swede." "We have no business to permit the perpetuation of citizens of the wrong type."

1904: The Station for Experimental Evolution, of the Carnegie Institution of Washington, DC, opens in Cold Spring Harbor, L.I., directed by biologist Charles Davenport and funded by Mary Harriman. It opens a Eugenics Records Office (ERO) in 1910 which becomes the epicenter of eugenics research on human inheritance that will provide scientific data to support the movement. ERO leaders propose that the "better" classes should be fruitful and multiply (positive eugenics) while "lower" classes should have their bad seeds literally cut off (negative eugenics.)

1905: Charles Davenport: "Heredity stands as the one great hope of the human race... The general program of the eugenicist is clear – it is to improve the race by inducing young people to make a more reasonable selection of marriage mates; to fall in love intelligently." Sterilization can "dry up the springs that feed the torrent of defective and degenerate protoplasm...The lowest stratum of society has neither intelligence nor self-control enough to justify the State to leave its mating in their own hands.... Death is nature's great blessing to the Race. Why keep defectives alive?"

1906: Dr. J.H.Kellogg (the breakfast cereal mogul) founds The Race Betterment Foundation in order to help stop the propagation of defectives. "Our race is going to seed...The world needs a new aristocracy...a real aristocracy made up of Apollos and Venuses and their fortunate progeny...the White Races of Europe [need] to establish a race of human thoroughbreds."

1907: Indiana is the first state to pass a law providing for government mandated sterilization. "Idiots, imbeciles and degenerate criminals are prolific and their defects are transmissible...So we owe it not only to ourselves but to the future of our race and nation to see that the defective and diseased do not multiply."

1907: Luther Burbank: "Only by selection of the best can any race be improved...Environment and education alone can not make appreciable progress in the improvement of the races. But with favorable surroundings and the selection of the best types, the field for improvement is limitless."

1909: Herbert Hoover: Black and Asian laborers should be avoided because they suffer from a "low mental disorder" and a pathological "lack of coordination and inability to take initiative...one white man equals two to three of the colored races."

1910: Winston Churchill supports segregation and compulsory sterilization for England's 120,000 feeble minded "so that their curse dies with them."

1912: Charles Darwin's son Leonard, presiding at the First International Eugenics Congress, extols eugenics as the practical application of the principle of evolution. The 20th century will be known as the time "when the eugenics ideal is accepted as the creed of civilization.... We shall conquer in time." However, implementation of better breeding procedures will require "moral courage."

1915: Irving Fisher (Yale economist): You have not any idea unless you have studied this subject mathematically, how rapidly we could exterminate this contamination [feeblemindedness] if we really got at it, or how rapidly the contamination goes on if we do not get at it."

1916: Madison Grant, a prominent conservationist, is more concerned with preserving Redwood trees and big game than human stock. His book *The Passing of the Great Race* is enormously influential. A white supremacist, he is called "the great patriarch of scientific racism." Eugenics policy promised to produce "a strong, virile and self contained race which would inevitably overwhelm nations whose weaker elements had not been purged." He notes that "the individual himself can be nourished, educated and protected by the community during his lifetime, but the state through sterilization must see to it that his line stops with him, or else future generations will be cursed with an ever increasing load of victims of misguided sentimentalism." Grant dehumanizes the feeble-minded calling them "human weeds or insects." The only really good group of humans are northern Europeans Nordics, except for the Irish.

1917: During World War I, Robert Yerkes, Louis Terman, Carl Brigham et al test the mental fitness of 1.7 million U.S. Army recruits and find that more than half meet Goddard's definition of morons; Jews 60%, negroes 86%. The "alpha" tests are biased in favor of scholastic skills and cultural background.

1920: Charles Davenport warns against "hordes of Jews" coming to America. Unless immigration is halted, Americans will have darker skin, grow smaller in stature and more emotional and become "more given to crimes of larceny, kidnapping, assault, murder, rape and sex-immorality." "Can we build a wall high enough around this country, so as to keep out these cheaper races?" If not, the Nordics will have "to abandon the country to the blacks, browns and yellows, and seek an asylum in New Zealand."

1922: Harry Laughlin of the ERO writes in *Eugenical Sterilization in the United States,* "The mothers of unfit children should be relegated to a place comparable to that of the female of mongrel strains of domestic animals." About eleven million Americans – "the lowest ten percent" – are unfit and are an economic and moral burden on the 90% -- "a constant danger to the national and racial life." They include paupers, drug addicts, the homeless, the blind or deaf, those with TB or syphilis.

1922: Lathrop Stoddard in *The Rising Tide of Color Against White World Supremacy: U*ncontrolled reproduction among defective families and the intermingling of defective and normal stock is causing "the twilight of the American mind" and "the dusk of mankind."

1923: Adolf Hitler reads Madison Grant's book and calls it his personal Bible: "Sentimental ideals about individual liberty must give way for the good of the people and in order to preserve the master race."

1923: Henry F. Osborn: "In the US we are slowly waking to the consciousness that education and environment do not fundamentally alter racial values. We are engaged in a serious struggle to maintain our historic republican institutions through barring the entrance of those unfit to share in the duties and responsibilities of our well-founded government…In the matter of racial virtues, my opinion is that from biological principles there is little promise in the melting-pot theory."

1924: President Calvin Coolidge signs the National Origins Act which limits influx of the "wrong types." Now no Asians are permitted in at all and other ethnic groups are limited to 2% of their total number present here as of the 1890 census. In effect, this closes "The Golden Door" so that by 1927 more people were being deported from Ellis Island than entering.

1926: The American Eugenics Society disseminates information to the public emphasizing that the dangerous and defective are reproducing too quickly, the normal and advantaged too slowly. They sponsor contests for "Fitter Families" at state and local fairs and, by now, eugenics is being taught at 75% of American colleges.

1927: Supreme Court Justice Oliver Wendell Holmes, Jr., in the *Buck v. Bell* decision upholds state sterilization practices: "It is better for all the world, if instead of waiting to execute degenerate offspring for crime, or to let them starve for their imbecility, society can prevent those who are manifestly unfit from continuing their kind." Referring to Carrie Buck's family: "Three generations of imbeciles are enough." The Court rules 8 to 1 to uphold the right of states to mandate sterilization of defectives against their wishes.

1933: Margaret Sanger declares that In order to create a decent civilization, a top priority is to rectify fertility imbalance through segregation or forced sterilization of severely feeble-minded persons. She coins the term "birth control" to limit the births of those who threaten the genetic integrity of humankind – it is "the most rational and efficient way to avoid race suicide." Sanger's motto is "More children for the fit; less for the unfit." "We need to breed a race of human thoroughbreds."

1936: Nobel Laureate Dr. Alexis Carrel (see previous chapter): "There is no escaping the fact that men are not created equal…the fallacy of equality was invented in the 18th century when there was no science to correct it…. Society must identify and encourage those with greatest ability, while the dregs should be disposed of in small euthanistic institutions supplied with the proper gases…Why preserve useless and harmful beings?"

1936: The University of Heidelberg awards an honorary degree to Harry Laughlin for his commitment to race purification which has inspired their own programs. An American eugenicist laments, "The Germans are beating us at our own game."

1941: Foster Kennedy, President of the American Neurologic Association: "The place for euthanasia, I believe, is for the completely hopeless defective: nature's mistake; something we hustle out of sight, which should never have been seen at all. These should be relieved of the burden of living…To allow them to continue such a living is sheer sentimentality, and cruel too; we deny them as much solace as we give our stricken horse. Here we may most kindly kill."

1942: Justice William O. Douglas in a case involving Oklahoma's compulsory sterilization law: "We are dealing here with legislation which involves one of the basic civil rights of man. Marriage and procreation are fundamental to the very existence and survival of the race. The power to sterilize, if exercised, may have subtle, far reaching and devastating effects…There is no redemption for the individual whom the law touches… He is forever deprived of a basic liberty." The Supreme Court stopped short of invalidating all compulsory sterilization, but by not overruling *Buck v. Bell* many more sterilizations were done during the next three decades.

1972: A Senate investigation finds that at least 2,000 sterilizations had been performed on poor black women without their consent or knowledge. Many were threatened with an end to welfare benefits until they consented. During this same period, more than 3,000 Native American women were coerced to consent to sterilization. By 1966, nationwide, about 65,000 people were involuntarily sterilized. Today sterilization laws remain on the books in twenty states.

OVERVIEW

Of course it is hazardous to apply today's standards to the past. Moreover, many people who used eugenics language didn't approve of the movement's most extreme negative agenda — all were not evil-minded or xenophobic racists. To be sure, most of them were elitists who wished to preserve a status quo which favored the affluent "fit" – like themselves. Among those who supported at least limited aspects of the eugenics agenda were Theodore Roosevelt, Woodrow Wilson, Warren Harding, Calvin Coolidge, Henry Ford, J.P. Morgan, Alexander Graham Bell, Thomas Edison, Abraham and Simon Flexner, Cecil Rhodes, G.B. Shaw, H.G. Wells, George Eastman, Clarence Gamble, Adolph Meyer, William Welch, Henry Sigerist, Alan Gutmacher, Charles Lindbergh, T.S. Eliot, Helen Keller and W.E.B. DuBois.

With The Great Depression at home and the rise of Fascism abroad, American and European society was restless. British geneticist J.B.S. Haldane warned that politicizing eugenics or enshrining it in law might unleash "the most ferocious enemies of human freedom." In this country nativism, economic hard times, fear of socialism and communism, anti-Semitism all contributed to a witch's brew of dissatisfaction. At the same time, there was a new progressive spirit with movements to reform education, focus on mental hygiene and prevent crime and poverty. With all of these cross currents and as scientific thinking was beginning to change, the balance between nature and nurture began to swing in favor of the latter. The utopian vision of eugenics gave way to a more critical perspective and more modest claims were made by former supporters.

Even conceding that the motives of most early eugenicists may have been well intentioned, events in Europe indicated that there could be unintended consequences. Nazi Germany used American laws as justification for compulsory sterilization of about 150,000 people; soon there were more than a million "mercy killings" and then mass murder. Even at the Nuremberg Trials after the end of World War II, American precedent was cited by Nazi defendants, as if to say, we were following your example. Although mandated sterilizations continued in many states during the 1940s, legal objections gradually began to gain the upper hand. Nevertheless, in California between 2006 and 2010 about 150 prison inmates were sterilized without informed consent.

According to historian Stephen Jay Gould (*The Mismeasure of Man*, 1981), "The eugenicists battled and won one of the greatest victories of scientific racism in American history. The paths to destruction are often indirect, but ideas can be agents as sure as guns and bombs." Eugenics did not evaporate after the Second World War – it transformed. In 1964 Mississippi lawmakers argued whether the state should arrest parents of illegitimate children (usually racial minorities) and offer them a choice of prison or sterilization. In 1998 an international survey of 2,901 geneticists in 36 nations suggested that eugenics thought underlies their perceptions of the goals of genetics. Although current practice promotes individual choice rather than state coercion and has shifted away from population concerns, the international survey concluded that "eugenics is alive and well."

In 1939 the Carnegie Institute concluded that work done by their Eugenics Research Office lacked scientific merit and withdrew funding. Soon the Cold Spring Harbor Laboratory transformed into a center of genetics research where eight Nobel Prize winners eventually would serve on its faculty. Nowadays the Laboratory's high-minded mission statement speaks of its dedication to molecular biology and curing diseases, but the word "eugenics" doesn't appear on its website. For nearly forty years the Laboratory was headed by James B. Watson, the co-discoverer of the structure of DNA, but when interviewed on BBC television in 2003, Watson employed eugenic rhetoric, speaking of getting rid of the lower 10%. It caused such furor that he was asked to resign.

With advances in biology and genetics there's been a revival of interest in the theory and practice of eugenics but this "new" eugenics claims to be different from the "old" oppressive eugenics - now it claims to be benevolent, voluntary, painless and efficient. Nonetheless, the "old" eugenicists considered themselves as having those very same qualities. The movement took quite different forms in different times and places and was promoted by individuals and groups with disparate social and political orientations, including progressives, environmentalists, peace activists, healthy living enthusiasts and decent family men and women. They thought of themselves as being kind and rational and if their positions were self-serving, they were justified as a scientific way of to prevent "race suicide" and promote human progress.

Today's scientists hope that with new techniques in the future they will be able to rewrite flawed genes in people, opening new possibilities for treating or even curing diseases. However, the boundary between healing and enhancing life is not easily demarcated. Tampering with genes in human embryos, eggs or sperm (already being attempted in China) raises the possibility of creating designer babies with enhanced intelligence, beauty or other traits – a fitter "master race" and all that implies. Perhaps the promise of genomics is being oversold but the dark history of the eugenics movement should give pause lest science is misused again for sinister purposes. Despite current excitement over the emerging field of genetics and its potential, the past history of eugenics should never be forgotten.

What really was wrong with Eugenics? Professor Diane Paul has suggested that the answer is far from obvious, that it depends on your point of view. In the narrow sense eugenics refers to the pre-World War II movement to reduce the "genetically unfit" and encourage breeding of the genetically advantaged. Certainly state coerced sterilization was repugnant and led to horrific results, but don't we practice a form of eugenics when we screen for Down's syndrome and other genetic abnormalities? Conventional thinking holds that the major distinction between the old and new eugenics is that the latter is based on choice. How about government mandated vaccinations for what is perceived as the greater good? Indeed many people today hold that everyone should have the right to pursue their own reproductive goals, that it's no business of the state to violate our privacy and that eugenic thinking reflects callous devaluing of certain people with disabilities.

With the benefit of hindsight, it's tempting to ask what were our ancestors thinking? A century from now will our descendants ask the same thing about us? Will they be shocked at some practices we feel to be perfectly correct? A dose of history-based humility is appropriate for, as Professor Paul concluded, "If the history of eugenics cannot provide straightforward lessons for policy, it does teach us that *neither* moralism nor complacency is justified." Exactly 100 years ago to this day (February 2, 1916), President Theodore Roosevelt, speaking to the National Americanization Committee, supported a proposed new law that would demand that new immigrants learn English and "live up to our ideals or be sent back home." The more things change, the more they are the same.

12. IMMIGRANTS

Most of what is contained in this chapter is extracted with permission from the unpublished memoir of Dr. Victor Parsonnet and from his family's archives that are housed at The Jewish Historical Society of New Jersey, Whippany, NJ.

In about 1890 two Jewish teenagers from what is now Ukraine arrived separately at Castle Gardens in lower Manhattan and eventually made their way to Newark, New Jersey where there was a large Jewish population. Neither 18 year old Victor Parsonnet (1871-1920) nor 17 year old Max Danzis (1873 -1953) could speak a word of English but within a decade both graduated from medical school, married and had children and were among a small group of recent immigrants who organized Newark's Beth Israel Hospital which opened in 1901.

After Czar Alexander II was assassinated in 1881, Jews were officially scapegoated and severe May Laws restricted their civil rights and educational opportunities. Government policy regarding Jews was described as one third starvation, one third assimilation and one third emigration. Victor's home city Balta (near Odessa) had a population of about 2,000, 80% Jewish, and a bloody pogrom there in 1892 spurred large scale Jewish emigration. But for Victor there was something else - as his son Eugene recalled, "father was a real revolutionary in his youth and had to escape Czarist Russia in order to save his life...It was a period of great love in this country; the streets were paved with gold [and] every mother's son could become President."

Shortly after landing in the New World Victor dropped his awkward Russian surname Petzetzelski in favor of Parsonett (later Parsonnet.) The choice may have been in honor of Albert Parsons, an American Socialist leader and anarchist who was hanged in 1887 following a bomb attack on Chicago police remembered as the Haymarket Riots. Indeed his son Eugene Victor Parsonnet was named for the famous Socialist leader Eugene Victor Debs. Victor (VP1) attended law school at Boston University for eighteen months before shifting to Tufts Medical College for another year and then transferring to Long Island Medical College Hospital from which he graduated in 1898. His wife Augusta Lavine ("Gusta") dropped out of medical school (LIMC) after two years because the couple couldn't afford two tuitions and went to work for the Singer Sewing Machine Company. She was public spirited and became a leading Suffragette in New Jersey and was active in the national movement.

Max Danzis was more descriptive than Victor about his early life:

> *I left Czarist Russia in my early youth because of the persecution and discrimination against the Jewish people. Conditions at that time were [in]tolerable, educational facilities, even of the most elementary type, were not extended to the masses and higher education was almost prohibitive to Jewish students. The doors of the universities were completely closed. Realizing that there was no future for me in Russia under such conditions, I determined, with the consent of my parents, to emigrate - America beckoned to me. Immigrants were welcomed here at that time. No obstacles were put in the way of immigrants who were seeking admission to the United States.*

Max Danzis was one of the first Jews to emigrate from Felshtin, a small shtetl in Podolia. (Information provided by the Felshtin Society indicates that "Mordsche Danzig," a 17 year old shoemaker arrived in New York from Antwerp on the *S.S. Rhynland* on July 11, 1890.) When he arrived with one ruble in his pocket, equivalent to about 50 cents today, Max lodged the first night in a stable and for much of the first year boarded with a *landsman* from Felshtin (Velvel Segal.) He worked by day as a delivery boy in a wrapping paper store at a salary of eight dollars a month and at night attended school and learned the language. In 1894 while working as a furrier in Manhattan he participated in a nationwide Hatters Strike. Within six years of coming to America Max Danzis obtained admission to Bellevue Hospital Medical College which in those days required only four years of high school. After graduating in 1899 he married Jenny Reich and most likely it was then that they settled in Newark where she may have had family. Little more is known about either of the two young men's early days but both were the first of their families to arrive in this country and once settled sent for relatives to follow them. And soon their lives would overlap in most significant ways.

Both Victor and Max worked extremely long hours as general practitioners and surgeons in Newark. In the early days the charge for a house call was one dollar, an office visit fifty cents, an obstetrical delivery twelve dollars, but many people couldn't pay anything and the burden of charity fell on the doctors' shoulders. At first Victor made house calls by horse and buggy, while going from floor to floor in a tenement sometimes seeing fifty patients in one building. Eugene Parsonnet recalled that when his father traded in the buggy for an automobile, he continued to carry a long whip so that when young boys hopped on the running board and yelled "get a horse, get a horse," he could beat them off! Later, Victor got a chauffeur to drive him around in his Ford or Reo. For his part, Max had a white horse called Joe whose black driver also was named Joe. Later both Joes were traded in for a Pierce-Arrow.

The Parsonnet and Danzis families lived close to each other in the Jewish section of Newark. Their first born children, Eugene Parsonnet and Rose Danzis, arrived within a few weeks of each other in 1900, grew up together and later married. Victor was a heavy cigarette smoker and died suddenly at age 49. About four years later Eugene and Rose married and when their son (VP2) was born August 29, 1924 he was named after his paternal grandfather. (A cousin Victor J. Parsonnet also was named after their mutual grandfather.)

Although VP2 never knew the man whose name he bore, Grandpa Max was a strong influence, both personally and professionally; remembered as "warm, cheerful, humble, a quiet leader, a voice of reason and a good listener." When Max graduated from the Bellevue Hospital Medical College (later NYU) in 1899, he was the first of four generations of the family to study there but, as VP2 has written, after his grandfathers settled in Newark they "sadly discovered that Jewish patients could not gain access to the local hospitals and Jewish doctors could not find staff appointments." There were two factions in the local Jewish community: one was a conservative element who didn't believe that a separate hospital was necessary and favored an ambulatory clinic (which opened in 1902.) However Victor and Max, both only recently arrived, were allied with a woman's organization, The Daughters of Israel, which in 1900 raised

$4,000 to purchase a three-story wood-frame house directly across West Kinney Street from the Parsonnet home-office.

The rival organizations merged in 1901 when the first Beth Israel Hospital opened with 21 beds; by 1908 with greater acceptance and a growing influx of Jewish immigrants, it expanded to new quarters with about 110 beds. The original staff consisted of twelve Jewish physicians - eight were very recent graduates - and 24 nurses. Within two decades the facility outgrew its early quarters and when philanthropists Louis Bamberger and Felix Fuld donated funds for a new non-sectarian hospital, it moved in 1928 to new facility which had 350 beds, a school of nursing and an outpatient building; the entire complex cost about $3.5 million.

Victor and Max spent their whole professional careers at Newark Beth Israel Hospital and served in various leadership roles both at the hospital and in the greater medical community. VP1 was sturdily built, vigorous, a dynamic personality, well informed on many subjects and active in progressive and socialist causes. He remained a political radical and in 1908 ran on the Socialist ticket for Alderman. Although Victor left no publications or speeches, eulogies praised his splendid surgical skill and devotion to patients. For his part, Max Danzis was responsible for the creation of new services - gynecology, obstetrics, orthopedics neurosurgery, ENT - and insisted that staff physicians qualify in their specialties. In about 1904 he was the first surgeon in New Jersey to perform a gall bladder resection and over the years he published and lectured widely on medical subjects. A former colleague (Henry Brodkin) once recalled Max as "our last angry man…always 'angry' at sham, pretentiousness, intellectual dishonesty and country club society." He was a student of medical history, particularly the part played by Jewish physicians since early times, and would astound groups of physicians with his erudition, frequently quoting from the Bible or the Talmud.

Max's wife Jenny helped acclimate immigrant women, teaching them useful trades such as sewing and organizing a cultural club to assist immigrants to acclimate themselves and learn English. In subsequent generations the family's influence on the hospital's development and culture was profound - among many family members who worked at Beth Israel were Victor's brother Aaron on staff for 45 years, his son Eugene for 66 years (1923-1966) and VP2 who joined his father's practice in 1955.

In March 1934 Dr. Danzis published a two part article "The Jew in Medicine" in *The American Hebrew and Jewish Tribune.* (Both in 1936 and 1941, together with Aaron Parsonnet, he reviewed the same subject in Newark's weekly newspaper *The Jewish Chronicle.*) Concerning the immigration of Russian Jews like himself to America during the late 19th century, Max wrote the following:

> *Included in this number was a large proportion of young men belonging to that group of Russian youth who threw off the yoke of narrow dogma and traditional Jewish ritualism. They were the ones who strongly yearned for more modern and higher education. They knocked at the portals of the higher educational institutions in Europe but were told that only a very small percentage of their number could be admitted.*

In this article, after reviewing Jewish contributions to medicine, Max discussed the results of a survey he conducted of the nation's 76 approved medical schools. He concluded that there was a national oversupply of doctors in numbers that was unequally distributed in relation to population size. Approximately 4,000 of the country's 22,000 medical students were Jewish, roughly 18%, which was more than five fold greater than other groups. Moreover, greater than 90% of American medical students studying in Europe were Jewish (1,173 in 1932.) Dr. Danzis found evidence of a quota system working against qualified Jewish applicants, especially in northeastern schools where after interviews students were denied entry on the basis of "ungentlemenly personality," deficient "magnetism" or absence of "professional inheritance." But his conclusion was discreetly worded: "I do not believe that there is a purposeful or coordinated effort on the part of all medical schools to restrict or limit the number of Jewish students but there is a tendency in many schools to keep them within a certain limited number."

However, there was something more urgent on Max Danzis' mind than the problems of American Jewish students. By the 1930s restrictive immigration laws had closed America's "Golden Door" to millions of East Europeans fleeing Nazi Germany and in 1938-39 all Jewish doctors in Germany were deprived of the right to practice. Max Danzis was one of five New Jersey physicians who joined a National Committee for the Resettlement of Foreign Physicians (later renamed the National Refugee Service.) The main purposes were to gather statistics and clarify misconceptions. (The other New Jersey members were Harrison Martland,

Edward Sprague, Henry Berkhorn and Royal Schaaf.) A less public object was to allocate immigrant physicians into underserved communities where there was need of more doctors and to prevent overcrowding in more desirable localities.

Between 1933 and 1940, more than 70% of some 5,000 immigrant physicians from Nazi Europe were Jewish; about 60% were able to receive licenses in fifteen states. Fearing competition, the Medical Society of New Jersey objected and in 1939 convinced the legislature to pass a law that all interns in the state had to be citizens; a law that was never enforced because the attorney general declared it to be unconstitutional. New Jersey was a medical wasteland located between New York and Pennsylvania with no medical school of its own and, because few American students wanted to train in the state, hospitals in Newark and Jersey City were especially dependent on immigrants and other foreign medical graduates as their primary source of interns. An undocumented source suggested that largely through the efforts of Dr. Danzis, 131 immigrants settled in New Jersey and he personally bore the expense of bringing many of them to safety. However, in his memoir VP2 noted that Grandpa Max "never spoke about the money - it was a topic that was shunned in the household, a vulgar subject."

On February 12, 1934 Max Danzis wrote a letter to Senator Kay Pittman of Nevada, Chairman (1933-1940) of the Senate's powerful Committee of Foreign Relations:

> *As an American citizen practicing surgery in New Jersey, being aware of the conditions taking place in Germany, with reference to discrimination against Jews and Jewish physicians particularly, I wish to express my sincere approval of your Resolution (154) and I appeal to you to use your influence with the Senate to have it approved.*

Immediately after Adolf Hitler's Nazi party assumed power in January 1933, they implemented anti-Semitic policies and now Chairman Pittman found himself in the middle of struggles between so-called "isolationists" and "internationalists." A proposal by Senator Millard Tydings called upon President Roosevelt to unequivocally condemn events in Germany but was blocked through the efforts of Secretary of State Cordell Hull. The feeling was that this was not our country's concern, that such an action would be embarrassing to the President and would prompt Germany to accuse us of hypocrisy - after all, Senator Tydings' home state of Maryland had been the scene of lynchings that were neither prevented or punished.

Undeterred, in January 1934 Senator Tydings introduced Resolution 154, which Dr. Danzis was writing to support. This time Tydings urged the Foreign Relations Committee itself, "as representatives of the people of the United States," to express their "profound feelings of surprise and pain upon learning of the discriminations and oppressions imposed by the Reich upon its minority groups, including its Jewish citizens [and to convey] its earnest hope that the German Reich will speedily alter its policy [toward Jews] and restore civil and political rights and undo the wrong that have been done them." Resolution 154 also died in committee. The next year the German government enacted the infamous Nuremberg Laws which institutionalized many of the racial theories that characterized Nazi ideology.

Sometime during the mid 1930s (the date is unclear), Max Danzis was honored by an organization that celebrated the contributions of foreign-born Americans. (His notes written on cue cards were discovered among his papers by VP2 only in 2013.) The following extracts from his acceptance speech seem particularly relevant today:

> *Mr. Chairman, honored Guests, fellow Immigrants:*
> *I deeply appreciate the honor that you are bestowing upon me this evening. I assure you that I am accepting it with a sincere feeling of humility. Awards of Meritorious Service always leave a lasting impression upon the recipient, even if the intent of the award far exceeds the individual's merit. After all, there is no special virtue in being helpful to your fellow-men. Civilized life would not have evolved without this human trait.*
>
> *If I may be permitted to say a few words about the early period of my life, I may summarize it by stating that my problems were common to all immigrants during the process of adaptation to a new environment. This is particularly true of those who belong to minority groups who were forced to emigrate from their homeland because of the denial of their civil rights. These people look hopefully to a land of tolerance and opportunity, a land which one of our early immigrants chose to call the "promised land."*

I must say that the process of adaptation to an entirely new condition of life is not an easy one for the immigrant even under the most favorable circumstances. Many find this period of struggle too hard to endure. Some take the road of least resistance and find it easier to travel with than against the stream. However, those who come here in the formative period of their lives bring with them ambition, enthusiasm, determination and an abiding conviction of ultimate success. To them these hardships act as a challenge to their ambition and a test of strength to their determination….

This has been aptly summarized by one of our American philosophers [Ralph Waldo Emerson] *in these words: "When Man is pushed, tormented, and defeated he has a chance to learn something, He has been put on his wits. He has gained facts, and is cured of conceit." I, as one who in the very early and most impressionable period of my life keenly felt the "rod of the persecutor", deeply appreciate living in a society where the rights and privileges of a human being, regardless of his religion, race or national origin, are held sacred.*

Whatever success I may have attained may be attributed to three main factors: 1. A Democratic country offering opportunities to all. 2. A state of society where a wide latitude is given to develop the trend of one's mental capacity or talent to the utmost of his ability. 3. The help and encouragement I received in molding my professional career from my wife who cheerfully shared and courageously bore with me all the hardships which we encountered in our early life. Her tireless interest in many social problems, such as adult education, health agencies and many others was really inspiring.

Most people are under the impression that life must be very hard for a young ambitious immigrant who has to earn his living at manual labor during his student days. That is not altogether true. Admitting that there are many physical hardships and inconveniences, there are also compensations. My most pleasant hours of the day during the years working at a bench were the evenings when I could retire in complete seclusion, away from the humdrum and sometimes the coarseness of a factory life, and become engrossed in my studies. On the surface one would think that I endured terrific hardships but I must say that all through these years, in spite of many difficulties, I never felt that life was hard. I had a goal in view. I had youth, I had ambition and foresight. Therefore, I looked forward to every evening which would bring me a step forward towards my educational goal.

I need not emphasize the responsibility of the immigrant to his adopted country. One of his main purposes and desires is to become a useful, dignified citizen and while the responsibility to the country of his adoption must be uppermost, nevertheless it is incumbent on him to be of help to those immigrants who come after him.

May I also at this point make a plea for more liberal immigration laws which are needed now. Tens of thousands of displaced persons who [were] kept in concentration camps through no fault of their own, men in all walks of life, some of whom were members of professional groups, are seeking refuge in new countries to rebuild their shattered lives.

Many social agencies stand ready to help these people not to become a burden on the public. With our immense territory and unlimited economic opportunities, it is safe to state that the admission of several hundred thousand immigrants would in no way interfere with or hinder the opportunities of our citizens.

As sons and daughters of immigrant groups, may I leave this thought with you. These displaced people need our help very badly.

On the occasion of Max Danzis' 75th birthday in 1949 and the 50th year since he entered the medical profession, Eugene Parsonnet lauded his father-in-law and former medical partner for his "rich, noble, gentle and genuine human life." The event was kept deliberately small affair befitting the modesty of the honoree:

Despite the heights to which he rose in his professional activity, he never lost his association and contact with simple folk. He never knew sham or pretense or guile. He never lost the common touch because he always stayed with, and was concerned with the lot of the humble, common man. Their problems were his. Their worries were his. Their hopes and plans for a better future were etched in his spirit and furnished both a guide and a goal for his life's work.

He never forgot - indeed he disdained - to cast from his mind or from his heart the reality of his early struggles, his early misfortunes. The hardships and handicaps of those early days became the basis and the cornerstone for his life's hope and ambition. Indeed, it developed into a crusade that the obstacles which had been his, and the difficulties which he was required to encounter and surmount should not prove to be a barrier to mar the life and work and ambition of eager and alert young men of another generation..... Dr. Danzis' mind, heart and spirit were all insistent that new avenues must be opened, in the democratic scheme of things, to furnish a full measure of opportunity for all aspiring, alert and eager young people who were touched by the fire for achievement and manifested the willingness to work.

It was with this basic concept...that he evolved and labored and toiled incessantly for the establishment of the Beth Israel Hospital which has now been for a generation a source of pride to our state and to the Jewish community. This hospital was Dr. Danzis' dream and the completion of the institution and its influence and importance were the result solely of his effort - a fact to which all of us here tonight can testify.

Dr. Danzis' story is the great American story. It is a story that bears repeating and reemphasizing. For his success, in the highest spiritual sense of the term, reflects the finest and noblest aspect of the American way of life.

When Max Danzis was named the recipient of the Award as the Outstanding Naturalized Citizen of Newark, New Jersey in 1950, he was hailed as "a foe of social, racial and religious bigotry, and an inspiring guide and benefactor to countless people in all walks of life...The story of Dr. Max Danzis is a realization of the American Dream and as such, reminds us that only if we practice the Golden Rule more fully, shall we approach the ultimate goal of democracy.... The Brotherhood of Man." And in 2000 when speaking at a dedication ceremony for the renamed Parsonnet/Danzis Auditorium, Victor Parsonnet observed that the narrative of his two grandfathers was typical of the lives and backgrounds of many of the founders of Newark Beth Israel Hospital. Virtually all were immigrants from Southeastern Russia and, although freed from persecution, "carried with them memories of what they left behind [and felt a need] to restore and improve upon a lost culture." They were passionate about "education, self-advancement, and service to all, regardless of origins or ethnicity and these principles [still] define the creed of the hospital to this day."

I'll let Max Danzis have the last word which, in effect, was his credo. Writing in 1934 he had prospective medical students in mind, regardless of their race or religion:

> *Medicine is a jealous profession. It demands a great many sacrifices from those who wish to join its ranks; and only those should join it who are capable and willing to place the higher value upon the opportunity for service to their fellow man and be ready to undergo many personal hardships. The medical student should be prepared to serve humanity in an altruistic manner; free from greed, selfishness and commercial tendencies....always ready to give cheerfully without any expectation of reward or public acclaim.*

13. THE FOOLMASTER

I once bought a thick well-worn book for a dollar at a local library sale that I thought was a standard 19th century medical text, but when I got home learned that it wasn't. The title page gave a hint why:

> *THE PEOPLE'S COMMON SENSE MEDICAL ADVISER IN PLAIN ENGLISH or, MEDICINE SIMPLIFIED. By R.V. PIERCE, M.D. One of the staff of consulting physicians and surgeons at the Invalids' Hotel and Surgical Institute, and President of the World's Dispensary Medical Association.*

My copy was the 20th edition and had been published in 1889 in Buffalo, N.Y. But the first edition appeared in 1875 and, in all, there were 80 editions with more than two million copies printed - available by mail order at $1.50 postpaid. The author's bearded face adorned the frontispiece followed by this grandiose dedication:

> *TO MY PATIENTS, who have solicited my professional services from their homes in every state, city, town, and almost every hamlet, within the American Union; Also to those dwellers in Europe, Mexico, South America, The East and West Indies, and other Foreign Lands.*

R.V. Pierce explained that the edition I bought was an entirely new rendition because "the popular favor with which former editions of this work have been received has required the production of such a vast number of copies that the original plates were worn out." And then came this:

> *That part of the book treating of Diseases and their Remedies will be found to be thoroughly reliable; the prescriptions recommended therein having well received the sanction and endorsement of medical gentlemen of rare professional attainments and mature experience.*

Distinguished physicians such as Austin Flint of Buffalo and Valentine Mott Jr. of New York City (son and namesake of a famous 19th century surgeon) were supporters. Indeed, in a letter to the editor of the *Journal of the American Medical Association* (Jan. 10, 1914, p. 146.) Dr. Mott had reported that he often used Pierce's panaceas both in hospital and private practice to treat "chronic syphilis, scrofulous complaints and obstinate cutaneous afflictions." No wonder that Dr. Pierce named his first born son Valentine Mott Pierce. Before discussing specific conditions, Dr. Pierce had some general observations which reflected his Victorian morality:

> *Although some of the subjects may seem out of place in a work designed for every member of the family, yet they are presented in a style which cannot offend the most fastidious, and with a standard avoidance of all language that can possibly displease the chaste, or disturb the delicate susceptibilities of persons of either sex.... We, as a people, are becoming idle, living in luxury and ease, and in the gratification of artificial wants. Some indulge in the use of food rendered unwholesome by bad cookery, and think more of gratifying a morbid appetite than of supplying the body with proper nourishment. Others devote unnecessary attention to the display of dress and a genteel figure, yielding themselves completely to the sway of fashion. Such intemperance in diet and dress manifests itself in the general appearance of the unfortunate transgressor, and exposes his folly to the world, with less precision than certain vices signify their presence by a tobacco-tainted breath, beer-bloated body, rum-emblazoned nose, and kindred manifestations. They coddle themselves instead of practicing self-denial, and appear to think that the chief end of life is gratification, rather than useful endeavor.*

Concerning the various sects or systems of medical practice: "old school," homeopathy, eclectic or "the liberal and independent physician," Dr. Pierce noted the following:

> *We do not deplore the fact that there are different schools in medicine, for this science has not reached perfection...We believe the time is coming when those maladies which are now considered fatal will be readily cured - when disease will be disarmed of its terrors. To be successful, a physician must be independent, free from all bigotry, having no narrow prejudices against his fellow-men, liberal, accepting new truths from whatever source they come, free from the restrictions of societies and an earnest laborer in the interests of the Great Physician.*

Following these introductory remarks came 920 pages of specific advice. In a section devoted to medications, Dr. Pierce touted his own *Golden Medical Discovery* claiming that it will "cleanse the blood, tone the system, increase its nutrition and establish a healthy condition." It would give men "appetite like a cowboy and the digestion of an ostrich." Even better were his *Pleasant Purgative Pellets* which promised to "awaken the latent powers, quicken the tardy functions, check morbid deposits, dissolve hard concretions, remove obstructions, promote depuration, harmonize and restore the functions, equalize the circulation, and encourage the action of the nervous system....[without] corroding the tissues or vitiating the fluids. Their assistance is genial, helping the system to expel worn out materials which would become noxious if retained." And if these weren't enough, one could order *Dr. Pierce's Anuric Tablets, Dr. Pierce's Smart-Weed* or *Dr. Pierce's Favorite Prescription.* In another chapter in his book, the doctor noted that "the remedial effects of baths are generally underrated" and described two dozen varieties - e.g. Russian, salt water, medicated, Sitz, douche. Best of all was the Turkish bath (dry, hot-air) which not only "combines a most agreeable luxury with a decidedly invigorating and tonic influence....Upon emerging the bather experiences a delightful sensation of vigor and elasticity." Naturally, Turkish baths were a therapeutic feature at The Invalid's Hotel.

Twenty-seven pages were devoted to the "degrading, polluting vice of masturbation" and its inevitable sequelae - spermatorrhea, impotency, nervousness and melancholy, enfeebled memory and intellect, softening of the brain, mania and insanity - "not a very uncommon result." Dr. Pierce moralized that "masturbation is a habit which tyrannizes over the mind, perverts the imagination, and forces upon the victim venereal desires." To break the habit he prescribed rising early, cold baths, cultivation of flowers, care of animals and such exercises as croquet, quoits and foot-ball. To drive his convictions home, Dr. Pierce provided forty-four case reports submitted by grateful patients, each attesting to the seriousness of their affliction and the wisdom of the doctor's advice. Then, on page 921, came "An Important Announcement."

> *Dr. R.V. Pierce, having in the Fall of 1880 resigned his seat in Congress, has since been able to devote his whole time and attention to the interests of the Association, and those consulting our Medical and Surgical Faculty have the full benefits of his counsel and professional services. That he should prefer to give up a high and honorable position in the councils of the nation, to serve the sick, is conclusive evidence of his devotion to their interests and of love of his profession.*

This was followed by 50 pages describing The Invalids' Hotel. A Model Sanitarium and Surgical Institute, staffed by 18 physicians and surgeons and "exclusively devoted to the treatment of chronic diseases…Not a hospital, but a pleasant remedial home" - now not only in Buffalo but also with a new branch in London, England. Next came a dozen testimonials for the institution, its leader and his book. The trustworthy *New York Times* enthused:

> *As a counselor and friend, DR. PIERCE is a cultured, courteous gentleman. He has devoted all his energies to the alleviation of human suffering, With this end in view and his whole heart in his labors, he has achieved marked and merited success. …The fact that there is a steadily increasing demand for his medicines, proves that they are not nostrums, but reliable remedies for disease.*

So who was Doctor R(ay) V(aughn) Pierce (1842-1914)? Certainly not a carnival huckster purveying snake-oil; in fact a Congressman elected to the State Senate in 1871, followed by a term as a United States House of Representatives. He received an MD degree from the Eclectic Medical College of Cincinnati in 1862 and five years later, after a brief fling at practice, moved to Buffalo where he opened his laboratory and distribution plant. Dr. Pierce was a marketing genius who promoted his products through newspaper ads, calendars, notebooks, billboards and barn sides. After the Pure Food & Drug Act passed in 1906, there was a major push to drive out hucksters. *Collier's* magazine published a series of articles titled

"The Great American Fraud" warning against patent medicines and quacks which the AMA reprinted and distributed as a pamphlet. When the *Ladies Home Journal* charged that one of Dr. Pierce's medicines contained liberal amounts of alcohol, quinine and opium, he sued for libel - and won. And when R.V. Pierce died in 1914, his son Valentine Mott Pierce continued the fight against government regulation and ran the family business until 1941 - their wondrous products still could be purchased by mail order as late as the 1970s.

By no means was R.V. Pierce the only successful purveyor of patent medicines during the late 19th century. Lydia Pinkham (1819-1883) was another shrewd marketer whose herbal-alcoholic "women's tonic" for menstrual and menopausal symptoms even outsold Pierce's remedies. However, the Buffalo doctor's approach had the aura of medical legitimacy. To be sure, Dr. Pierce was merely a successful exponent of a time-honored tradition of self-promoters who excelled in deceiving the public.

Historian James Harvey Young of Emory University began his analysis "The Foolmaster Who Fooled Them" (*The Yale Journal of Biology and Medicine* 53 (1980), 555-566) by citing a paragraph from Owen Johnson's novel *Stover at Yale* (1912):

> *One evening at Mory's, Dink Stover sits listening to Ricky Rickets discourse on how he plans to become a "millionaire in ten years." That certain route to wealth lies in "making an exact science" of beguiling the foolish. "What's the principle of a patent medicine?" Ricky asks rhetorically, and then answers himself: "[A]dvertise first, then concoct your medicine." All the science of Foolology," he elaborates, "is: first, find something all the fools love and enjoy, tell them it's wrong, hammer it into them, give them a substitute and sit back, chuckle, and shovel away the ducats. Why, Dink, in the next twenty years all the fools will be feeding on substitutes for everything they want; no salt — denatured sugar — anti-tea—oiloline—peanut butter—whale's milk—et cetera, et ceteray, and blessing the name of the* ***foolmaster*** *who fooled them.*

Professor Young noted that in his 1850 essay "Lessons from the History of Medical Delusions," Worthington Hooker had sought to expose the methods of "foolology," explained why it flourished and condemned its results. He declared, "This an age of nostrums,…they are as abundant and clamorous as were the frogs in one of the plagues of Egypt, when they came croaking into the houses and even the bedchambers." Newness and secrecy, when attributed to nostrums, lent them allure. A "high-sounding name" or slogan enhanced its stature, such as *Dr. Sweet's Infallible Linament* or *Goelicke's Matchless Sanitize - the Very conqueror of Physicians."*

Professor Young noted that quackery flourished not only because of the cleverness of charlatans and the gullibility of the masses for other groups shared in the guilt:

> *These included the "old aunt Betsies" of the community gossiping the neighbors into trying nostrum brands; the lords of the press who accepted the nostrum-makers' fees despite the social dangers in their medical messages; the clergy, who often blundered into praising nostrums, thus imbuing them with a dimension of faith healing. And receiving especially severe rebukes from physician critics were their own erring brethren who in various ways, witting and unwitting, encouraged unorthodoxy.*

Professor Young despaired that we haven't progressed as much as we like to think since the 19th century and noted that the annual bill for unproven arthritis remedies approximates a half billion dollars while the tab for irregular cancer treatments might exceed that.

> *The bill for unorthodox nutrition is higher still and soaring. Sects like chiropractic and naturopathy, the basic rationales of which scientific medicine has rejected as naive flourish widely. Homeopathy now is reviving.... A massive effort has been made in our day...to make alternative therapies to scientific medicine seem like the legitimate road to health, whereas scientific medicine is decried as wrong and dangerous, its practitioners not only blind but money mad. Legitimate self-criticism from within orthodox medicine's own ranks, such as charges that some physicians improperly prescribe or overprescribe today's powerful medicines, can, of course, be turned to good effect in the propaganda of the unorthodox.*

Writing nearly four decades after Professor Young, I can't see that we've advanced much.

14. ODDBALLS, QUACKS & CONMEN

R.V. Pierce was by no means unusual in his time and what follows next is adapted from a lecture I gave at The Learning Collaborative, Orangeburg, NY in 2015.

Medical healers weren't always good guys in white coats. There has always been a parallel universe of bad guys who, at least metaphorically, wore black coats. They included a mélange of charlatans, snake oil peddlers and outright scoundrels. The public didn't care about sectarian squabbles between orthodox practitioners and popular healers — it was results that mattered. At mid-19th century The Medical Society of New Jersey reported there were 596 "Regulars" and 151 (20%) "Irregulars" practicing in the state. The Irregulars included 60 homeopaths, 36 "eclectics," 6 Thomsonians, 5 Botanicals, 6 "electricians," 5 cancer doctors, 5 clairvoyants, 3 root doctors, 2 of the "Swedish Movement," 2 hydropaths, 1 Indian doctor and 1 inhalation practitioner. Two more were listed simply as "Quacks" and 17 were not classified or practiced no particular system. 21 of the 151 "irregulars" were women who were described as "of the class known as the progressive bloomer kind, infidels and spiritualists."

This last category of spiritualists had a particularly devoted clientele although usually not because of their medical treatments. Their main purpose was to communicate with the dead through séances conducted by mediums. The unlikely founders of the movement were **The Fox Sisters**, two teenagers who lived in Hydesville, a small hamlet in Upstate New York about 20 miles west of Rochester. During the 1840s the sisters became widely known as "The Rappers" and it all began with a prank when 15 year old Maggie and her eleven year old sister Katy wanted to scare their mother. They began making noises at night suggesting that the farmhouse was haunted – noises so loud that they woke their parents up. Then the girls developed a way of snapping the tendons in their feet – like cracking your knuckles – and became so adept that they could make loud noises even with their shoes on. Their mother put the spirits to the test by asking questions and the girls would rap back an answer – once for yes, twice for no. Mrs. Fox called in the neighbors, word spread and, before long, spiritualism became a national and then an international phenomenon. The Fox sisters were afraid to admit their trickery and enjoyed the attention. Accounts of their prowess made them rural super-stars and their stories became more and more elaborate. In 1850 an older sister was recruited, and now the three Foxes began giving public exhibitions and private seances.

The esteemed Professor Austin Flint (who'd recently founded the nearby Buffalo Medical College and later became President of the AMA) was consulted and with two colleagues made a special investigation. Their official report concluded that it was all a hoax – the "rapping" sounds could be induced by moving various joints to snap tendons. The Fox sisters confessed but soon recanted. As one explained, "It was such a comfortable easy way of making a living and it was such good fun to pit one's wits successfully against those of the investigators who came so confident of their ability not to be fooled." Although the sisters were exposed as false mediums, spiritualism and its variants spread throughout the civilized world and before long every town had a regular circle of "inquirers." More than a hundred periodicals were devoted to news of the spiritual world and during the 1870s, despite a series of exposures of mediums everywhere, there were more than enough dupes ready to believe them. The fact that credible scientists were unable to explain the "miracle cures" underscored the belief that supernatural factors must be at work.

In Chicago during the early 20th century, Dr. **Ben Reitman** (1879--1942) earned a reputation as a whorehouse physician and eccentric; Studs Terkel called him "Chicago's most eminent clap doctor." Reitman was friend and physician of scores of Al Capone's prostitutes and his clientele included drifters, dope addicts, hustlers and pimps -- society's refuse. Born in Minnesota to poor Russian immigrants, his father and grandfather were itinerant peddlers which may have contributed to his life-long wanderlust. He left home at age 12 to ride the rails, lived in Hobo "jungles," slept in YMCAs or haystacks and learned to mooch handouts and steal food. He ran with a rough crowd – most of them very young, under age 21. Consider the names of some of Ben's buddies: *Ohio Skip, Jerusalem Slim, Sailor Bill, Dopey Liz, Chinatown Blinky, Gloomy George, Hot Tamale Kelly, John the Joker, One Tooth Scully, Olaf the Unwashed, Pessimistic Bernheimer, Flat-Head Horatio, Pittsburgh Spider Leg.* Ben Reitman was known as the *Chi Kid* and sometimes described himself as a Master Bum. He believed that many of these homeless punks, beggars and tramps had a certain nobility – he called them "knights of the rails" - and were more victims than villains. But polite society considered these outcasts to be products of their own moral inadequacies – after all, jobless men and women could find employment if they really wanted to.

Ben Reitman's medical education wasn't exactly conventional. As a teenager he worked briefly as a janitor in a medical laboratory in Chicago and impressed his bosses by his diligence. One of them, Dr. Leo Loeb (who many years later became famous for being the first to treat endocarditis with penicillin and heparin) hired the bright young man from the slums as a pathology assistant and offered to pay for his medical school tuition. Despite his virtual lack of education, Ben entered med school in 1900 and in order to pay for text books, sold stray dogs and cadavers to his classmates so they could practice their surgical skills. He nearly got married but left the bride at the altar and fled to Europe where he bummed around for a while before returning on a tramp steamer to resume school. Somehow he graduated in 1904 from the American College of Medicine & Surgery (later Loyola), obtained a license and opened an office in the red light district. His patients included pimps, prostitutes, pickpockets and perverts. In his off-duty time he caroused and gambled, yet, somehow, he also found time to teach a few courses about VD at local medical schools and working with Chicago's authorities during the 1930s he established a Society for the Prevention of Venereal Disease.

Whenever the routine became too confining he'd close the office and hit the rails – or hop a tramp steamer for Mexico or Manchuria. In Paris he joined Buffalo Bill's Wild West show and treated the circus hands for VD. Back in Sin City (Chicago) in 1906, with a few like-minded sinners, he started a Hobo College which was a center for education, political organizing and social services for migrants. The disheveled students studied economics, astronomy, philosophy and poetry as well as more practical subjects about the current status of "trampdom" -- e.g. how to survive on the road, which towns were most or least welcoming, how to survive without eating regularly. The Hobo College also promoted the arts. The acclaimed opera star Mary Garden sang at one of their concerts in Hobo Hall and famous writers and intellectuals participated in public debates in which the students easily held their own. They had their own monthly newspaper called *The Hobo News* (1815--1829) and Ben always provided wonderful copy for the conventional press which brought him fame and notoriety – the journalists dubbed him the "King of the Hoboes." He always was a soft touch and liberally handed out nickels and dimes whenever he was panhandled.

In his early years, Doc Reitman was an imposing if shabby figure – tall and self-assured, he had bushy hair and a black mustache, wore a large cowboy hat, usually dressed in a cape and flowing silk tie and carried a large walking stick. He was a life-long womanizer to the dismay of his three wives and his famous lover the anarchist Emma Goldman. In fact, Emma was a good influence and smoothed off some of his rough edges. Ben organized and spoke at her rallies and for six months in 1916 they spent time in jail together for violating the Comstack laws by advocating birth control. Through Emma Goldman's influence, Doc developed a passion for progressive ideas -- including woman's rights, abortion and birth control. But although both believed in free-love, Emma couldn't abide his womanizing and they broke up after nearly a decade on the road together. As Ben once described himself:

> *I am an American by birth, a Jew by parentage, a Baptist by adoption, single by good fortune, a physician and teacher by profession, cosmopolitan by choice, a Socialist by inclination, a rascal by nature, a celebrity by accident, a tramp by twenty years' experience, and a tramp reformer by inspiration.*

Ben Reitman considered himself a born anarchist: "I was always against things – sometimes I was even against myself." But by the 1930s the fire had gone out, the world had moved on and in 1942 he died of a heart attack at age 63. This is how his biographer remembered him:

> T*he man left his mark…not only in the annals of bombast and crudity, but as one of America's most colorful reformers. He left his mark in the hearts of numerous outcasts, from the joyladies in Chicago, to the hoboes to the bohemian philosophes. He also left his mark as one of the country's most spirited, if unorthodox, radicals.*

At least Ben Reitman had a legitimate medical license. That wasn't the case with **John Romulus Brinkley** (1885-1942) from tiny Milford, Kansas who during the 1920s and 30s was the country's most notorious medical huckster. He bought a medical school diploma for $500 from the Eclectic Medical University (R.V. Pierce's alma mater) which allowed him to obtain a license to practice in several Western states. He soon became public enemy number one for the AMA's leader Morris Fishbein who, like a medical version of Inspector Javert of Les Miserables, pursued phony doctors on his personal crusade to rid the country of charlatans. But for two decades this nimble flim-flam man kept two-steps ahead of the law -- and the AMA. The more critics he attracted, the greater was his appeal to the unwashed masses who fancied him as the people's doctor. No matter that he had a phony diploma. Although he grew up dirt poor in rural Kansas he lived like a prince and became one of the country's wealthiest men; among his close friends of the international set were the Duke and Duchess of Windsor. Doc and his wife sailed the world's oceans in their three yachts; they had airplanes, multiple houses and a fleet of Cadillacs. His name flashed in neon lights outside his largest mansion and the swimming pool was adorned with swastikas in honor of The Fuehrer whom he admired. None of this troubled his faithful fans.

And what was the basis of Brinkley's phenomenal success? Goat testicles! Glandular rejuvenation was an international craze during the late 19th and early 20th century. The famous French physician Charles Brown-Sequard had injected crushed testes of young dogs and guinea pigs into himself and claimed to feel more virile. Then his colleague Serge Voronoff transplanted the testicles of young lambs into aging rams, reported impressive results and developed a thriving practice. It was time for someone to do the same in this country. Starting in 1917, the so-called "Ponce de Leon of Kansas" began reporting that goat glands worked wonders on 27 different ailments from dementia and emphysema to flatulence and acne. Patients would come to his hospital and choose the goat that they fancied from his flock. It was castrated on the spot, the implant took only a few minutes and the placebo effect kicked in soon afterward. Doc Brinkley didn't actually bother attaching the goat testicles, but merely dropped them into a slit he made in the recipient's scrotal sac where he claimed they spontaneously "humanized." He promised to make every man "the ram that am -- with every lamb." After some 16,000 testicular "transplants", he modestly claimed only a 95% success rate – although the failures included several hundred deaths these were ignored. He had trouble keeping up with the demands for glands even though the price was high; on average he charged $750 for goat testes and a minimum of $5,000 for the human variety which he bought from prisoners on death rows. For lesser conditions and for a small fee of only $25 he'd inject distilled colored water wherever it hurt, but although he soaked the rich, this medical Robin Hood didn't give back to the poor -- there were no freebies. If you were nearly destitute you could mail order a Special Gland Emulsion for only $100 which could be self-administered through a rectal syringe.

Doc Brinkley shamelessly promoted himself on his own radio station which was beamed all over the country from his home base in rural Kansas. When federal authorities closed his station on the grounds that it was promoting fraud and immorality, Doc set up the world's most powerful transmitter just over the Mexican border and continued broadcasting. He may have been the first to use radio advertising, promoting not only his own wares but any kind of patent medicine or fraudulent cure that others would pay him to air. A popular feature on his radio station was The Medical Quiz Box in which people would call in their ailments. Doc diagnosed them sight unseen and then sold the sufferers unnamed drugs at exorbitant prices. His medical advice was accompanied by soothing homilies and hillbilly music and the so-called "Milford Miracle Man" or "Milford Messiah" was a sensation!

When government watchdogs got too close for comfort he decided to join them and twice ran for governor of Kansas, narrowly losing when establishment politicians fixed the votes against him. Doc was the first politician to fly in his own airplane from place to place spreading his message of rejuvenation and redemption. Undaunted by his defeat for governor, he considered a run for president but his grandiosity didn't end there -- he likened himself to Jesus, beset and betrayed, and took to evangelism. In one sermon he said, "I had rather save a soul than be President of the United States or even King of the World."

Although the AMA's Morris Fishbein collected reams of testimony about disasters and deaths, gullible patients and wealthy patrons were delighted to submit testimonials. But the more evidence gathered to expose him, the better Brinkley thrived. Inevitably the AMA and the law caught up with the Doc -- his licenses were revoked, his station closed down, there were law suits for wrongful deaths, tax-evasion, mail fraud, his lavish possessions were seized and he was forced into bankruptcy. But when Doc Brinkley died in May 1942, even his fiercest critics grudgingly acknowledged his genius. The AMA's Morris Fishbein said, "The centuries to come may never produce such blatancy, such fertility of imagination, and such ego." Journalist William Allen White wrote, "What a little tinkering with his character might have done…A [little] more honesty here, a little more intelligence there…would have made him a really great leader of men."

15. SEXOLOGY

Prepared for a Medical History Society of New Jersey conference held at The Belskie Museum in Closter, NJ, May 31, 2014.

Charles Knowlton (1800-1850) financed his medical education at Dartmouth Medical School by grave robbing! That was not uncommon in early 19th century America. He sold bodies to the school's anatomy department for $50 apiece - an enormous sum in those days - and in 1834 boldly wrote in his senior thesis (see chapter 6) about a need for laws to be passed which would encourage people to willingly donate their own bodies. Knowlton's last words contained an interesting proposal:

> *Let it become a general practice for physicians to give their bodies by will, for dissection and the prejudice existing on the subject will soon be done away; and it will be as common for persons to request that their bodies may be dissected, as it now is, for them to beg that their graves may be guarded against resurrectionists* [grave robbers.]

At Dartmouth's Commencement when Professor Reuben Mussey told the young man, "You have done our Institution great honor," apparently he wasn't aware that at the very same time Knowlton was under indictment in Massachusetts having been arrested the previous summer for "illegal dissection." Indeed, after receiving his Dartmouth diploma, the fledgling doctor spent two months in jail and his father was obliged to pay a $284 fine. That was lenient because the penalty for grave robbing in New Hampshire earlier in the 19th century was a $2,000 fine, two years imprisonment, "setting on the gallow" and 50 lashes!

Charles Knowlton was a free thinker and an outspoken agnostic; neither were popular positions in western Massachusetts where he set up practice after graduation. When his book *The Fruits if Philosophy. The Private Companion of Young Married People,* appeared in 1832, its anonymous author was listed only as "A Physician." This manual was a treatise on the medical and social aspects of birth control and in the first five years sold some 7.000 copies. Priced from fifty cents to one dollar, it was kept deliberately high to keep it out of the hands of minors. Knowlton's recommended douching after conjugal relations either with water or a "vegetable astringent" via a vaginal syringe. He argued that this was a "sure, cheap, convenient and harmless method, which should not in any was interfere with enjoyment." One chapter heading promised "to show how desirable it is, both in a political and social point of view for mankind to be able to limit at will the number of their offspring without sacrificing the pleasure that attends the gratification of the reproductive instinct." For his efforts Dr. Knowlton was fined $50 for publishing an obscene book and sentenced to three months hard labor in Cambridge. But undaunted, he continued to promote his ideas and his work drew national and then international attention; female syringes were sold in all apothecary shops and when the book was republished in England in 1877 it became a *cause celebre* as much over the legal issue of free speech as the personal matter of birth control.

About a century after Charles Knowlton's sex manual appeared, a Brooklyn gynecologist **Robert Labou Dickinson** (1861-1950) published *Human Sex Anatomy*, an atlas with 174 of his own illustrations of the genitals including during intercourse.

Dr. Dickinson was born in Jersey City and while still a young child his prosperous father took the family to Europe on a vacation that lasted four years. Upon their return in 1876 when they moved to Brooklyn Heights he had a serious canoeing accident, an experience which influenced him to become a doctor. After completing medical studies at Long Island College Hospital in 1880, he had to wait a year until he was 21 before he could get a license, and because he had a talent for drawing, spent the time off working as an illustrator for a textbook of gynecology which would become a classic. The author was Alexander Skene, a prominent Brooklyn physician who encouraged his students to specialize in gynecology and, in due time, young Dr. Dickinson developed a busy practice which lasted for about forty years. Although generally an orthodox practitioner, Dickinson was distinctly unusual for his time when it came to questioning and counseling his patients about sex and contraception. He recorded detailed sexual histories of his married patients which were accompanied by his sketches and eventually these amounted to more than 5,200 records.

Dr. Dickinson persuasively promoted his ideas at medical meetings and in 1920 he successfully lobbied to become president of the American Gynecological Society. In his inaugural address he criticized colleagues for their insufficient interest in the medical aspects of sexuality. He retired from practice at age sixty, lived off his investments and moved to Manhattan where he set up an office at The Academy of Medicine. He launched a "second career" as a promoter of sex research and marriage counseling and dared to publicly advocate contraception. In 1923 he founded The Committee on Maternal Health which promoted a broad program to improve the quality of life" by liberating married women from disease, disability and ignorance - as he said, sex was "a force to be accepted and enjoyed…children should be wanted, planned and spaced." When his atlas *Human Sex Anatomy* appeared in 1933 it was lambasted as pornography but, undaunted, in 1937 he convinced the conservative AMA, which fancied itself as a defender of "civilized morality," to endorse contraception as a legitimate medical service and to encourage the teaching of sexology in medical schools. This despite the objections of the AMA's opinionated leader Morris Fishbein who asserted that "there is no method of birth control that is physiologically, psychologically or biologically sound in both principle and practice."

The Comstock Act, a federal law passed shortly after the Civil War (1873) banned sending obscenity through the mails - not only pornography but also contraceptives and contraceptive advice. But in 1915 Margaret Sanger (1879-1966), a headstrong nurse defied Anthony Comstock's "Society for the Suppression of Vice" by importing diaphragms from Europe and Japan and when she couldn't find a single New York City doctor to fit pessaries, did it herself in a clinic she set up in Brooklyn. After ten days the police shut the clinic down and Sanger fled the country to avoid prosecution. But she had powerful allies, including the anarchist Emma Goldman and her lover "The Hobo King" Ben Reitman (see previous chapter) and socialists like John Reed and Eugene Debs. When the tumult died down Sanger returned and resumed her campaign for what she called "a woman's right to birth control." Her slogan was that women should raise more hell and fewer babies. Progressive European influence was making inroads on American prudishness thanks to the writings of Sigmund Freud and Havelock Ellis among others and in 1936 the Comstock Act was overthrown by the courts.

Margaret Sanger and Robert Labou Dickinson had an on-again, off-again relationship, sometimes rivals, other times collaborators, and disagreeing over who should control reproduction - the women themselves (MS) or their doctors (RLD.) There also was a dark side to their similarities since both were ardent eugenicists. The term "eugenics," meaning "good birth," had been coined in 1883 by Charles Darwin's brilliant cousin Francis Dalton and many intellectuals were advocates - the likes of Teddy Roosevelt, Winston Churchill, Woodrow Wilson, Alexander Graham Bell, George Bernard Shaw, Norman Thomas and Alexis Carrel. Both Dickinson and Sanger supported the eugenics agenda for forced sterilizations, justifying social engineering both on the basis of religious morality and on Darwinian principles. They viewed contraception as a tool to preserve the American way of life; Sanger's slogan was "More children for the fit; less for the unfit." According to her, the latter included "Hebrews, Slavs, Catholics and negroes." To be sure, feminists like Sanger were less enthusiastic about so-called "positive eugenics" - after all, more babies by the fit would further enslave women to the traditional role of homemaker.

During his last years, Dr. Dickinson went to California to learn what was being done in the state where more sterilizations were performed than in the rest of the world combined. He encouraged a technique of intrauterine cauterization which would render women infertile but not lessen their pleasure, perhaps even enhancing it - as he described, "sterilization without unsexing." He debunked various myths about copulation and masturbation and supported the use of a new German invention - an intrauterine device to prevent contraception. He also advocated the use of vibrators and genital stimulation by doctors during pelvic examinations of frigid women in order to release damaging sexual tension. Dickinson also advocated "mercy killing" and as late as 1948 still was defending Nazi policies of premarital testing and euthanasia as a way of eliminating hereditary disorders.

In 1943 Dr. Dickinson joined an organization called "Birthright" which was the brainchild of a feisty Princeton social worker Marian Olden. Like Margaret Sanger, Olden believed that the best breeding stock should be encouraged to be fruitful and multiply; the rest literally cut off from their ability to reproduce. The organization underwent several metamorphoses and although Dickinson and Olden often didn't agree, he eventually became it's vice president. Also in 1943, Dickinson met a young biologist from Indiana who would succeed him as the country's leading sexologist, Legend has it that when Alfred C. Kinsey first met Robert Latour Dickinson, the old man tearfully exclaimed, "At last! At last! This is what I've been hoping for all these years." In turn, the younger man acknowledged his debt to Dickinson which included receiving all of his research data. In 1946 Dickinson won the prestigious Lasker Award for career contributions as "America's leading medical sexologist." This was two years before Kinsey's first book appeared and when Dickinson received his copy, he wrote to the man whom he called ACE, "I have my copy at last. Glory be to God." Everyone didn't agree and when Kinsey published his first books in 1948 and 1952, they elicited enormous criticism of perceived pornography, similar to what befell Dickinson's book in 1933 and Charles Knowlton's in 1832.

16. NEW JERSEY'S HALLS OF MEDICAL FAME AND SHAME

Text for 12th annual Allen Weisse Lecture delivered at Rutgers New Jersey Medical School, September 29, 1915.

In 2013 at one of our semi-annual meetings in Princeton, as president of the Medical History Society of New Jersey, I invited all those present to choose from a preselected list what they felt were the *most important medical events* in our state's history. The poll was flawed in many respects — thoroughly unscientific, totally subjective and certainly not intended to be taken seriously. Nevertheless, the results provided a snapshot of the opinions of a varied group who at least shared enthusiasm for local medical history.

Although our survey may have been the first of its kind, over the years several books had been written about New Jersey's medical history. The first one by Dr. Stephen Wickes in 1879, described several prominent physicians during Colonial times. During the 1960s, our late colleague Professor David Cowen, regretted that Wickes chose not to cover the 19th century and wrote his own classic *Medicine and Health in New Jersey: A History.* In 2002 historian Karen Reeds published *A State of Health: New Jersey's Medical Heritage* and for its bicentennial in 1966, the Medical Society of New Jersey published *The Healing Art* which listed many names and events. One of its co-authors, Fred Rogers also had written an earlier book (1960) *Help-Bringers. Versatile Physicians of New Jersey* which provided vignettes about a dozen pre-20th century doctors and I'll briefly mention just two of them in order to give the old-timers their due.

One was **William Augustus Newell** (1817-1901) who graduated from Rutgers in 1836 and then earned his medical degree at the University of Pennsylvania. In addition to practicing medicine, he was active in politics and as a member of the House of Representatives was responsible for passing an act to create a Life Saving Service along the New Jersey coast which later became the US Coast Guard. Dr. Newell was both friend and physician of Abraham Lincoln's family and in 1847 he became New Jersey's 23rd governor (1857-1860.) Apparently these credentials didn't impress the Monmouth County Medical Society which in 1881, on the advice of their ethics committee, censured Dr. Newell for what they described as "an indiscretion, to say the least." And what was that? He was found guilty of consulting with herbal practitioners and other so-called "irregulars" which conflicted with the AMA's strict code of ethics that banned collaboration with the enemy. After being censured by the Medical Society, Dr. Newell went west and served for several years during the 1880s as governor of the Washington Territories. During his last years the former governor returned to New Jersey where he died penniless in 1901. Certainly a varied career with highs and lows.

Another 19th century notable was **Ezra Mundy Hunt** (1830-1894) of Metuchen whose experiences during the Civil War impressed him with the importance of hygiene to control epidemic diseases. After the war he became president of New Jersey's medical society and was a national pioneer in the public health movement. When the state legislature anticipated an impending cholera epidemic, it formed a Sanitary Commission with Dr. Hunt as its chief. Later, he was instrumental in organizing New Jersey's Department of Health and in that capacity promoted mass vaccination and waste removal and insisted upon accurate data collection about the incidence of disease in different locations. When Dr. Hunt attended a national AMA meeting in 1870, he was dismayed that there was organizational bias against colored delegates and reported back to his New Jersey colleagues that, in his opinion, anyone with "certified competency and character" should be admitted to membership: "We have enough to do to contend with the irregularities of pretense and quackery and false creeds of doctoring without drawing ethnological distinctions." With no medical school of its own, New Jersey was considered to be a medical backwater, but Dr. Hunt disagreed and had this to say when writing to a colleague in 1888:

> *There is no medical wilderness between New York and Philadelphia. We can name scores of members of this Medical Society who from 1875 on, have kept well-informed as to the prominent and popular medical hypothesis of the period and have given it consideration in their study and treatment of disease.*

Note that he said "from 1875 on", not from 1775 on for, no doubt, he was referring to the recent work of Pasteur and Koch. Nevertheless, Dr. Hunt admitted that the greatest barriers to hygienic reform existed within the medical profession itself which still was concerned, almost exclusively, with curing rather than preventing disease.

Enough about the really old old-timers so now let's consider the results of our history society's survey. I'm sure that some will protest "How could you leave out Dr. so and so?" And I don't want to offend any living people so please indulge me. I'll begin with two events that weren't identified with any particular individual physician or scientist. The leader in this category, with seven votes out of a possible twenty three, was the New Jersey Supreme Court's decision in 1976 concerning the tragic case of **Karen Ann Quinlan.** Not only did their ruling profoundly impact how end-of-life decisions are made but, in some respects, altered the dynamic between doctors and patients — favoring patient autonomy over traditional physician paternalism. The Quinlan case drew worldwide attention and discussions of Karen's fate introduced such terms into our vernacular as "death with dignity," "pulling the plug" and "a right to die." It surely was the most influential single case in New Jersey's history and the Court's opinion became a legal landmark which set the stage for later decisions, such as the famous cases of Nancy Cruzan and Terri Schiavo. In our survey there were three votes for another once famous medical event that occurred here in Newark in 1885 when four Newark school boys were bitten by a rabid dog. They were sent to Paris to receive Pasteur's brand new rabies vaccine, it caused a national media sensation and money was raised from all over to send the boys abroad. With those two events as preliminary, here were the top individual vote getters in our thoroughly unscientific survey in reverse order.

New Jersey is famous for its pharmaceutical industry with much outstanding research done here by tens of thousands of laboratory scientists. One important contributor was a Croatian born chemist **Leo Sternbach** (1908-2005) who is credited with discovering benzodiazepine tranquilizers, including Librium and Valium. During the 1930s he worked for Hoffman-La Roche in Switzerland, but in 1941 fled to this county to escape the Nazis. Working at the Roche plant in Nutley, Dr. Sternbach held more than 240 patents which helped make the company into an industry giant although he didn't personally become wealthy as a result of his discoveries. In 2003, on the 40th anniversary of Valium's approval, the 95 year old scientist told *The New Yorker* that it was a very good drug, adding: "It has pleasant side effects. It's quite a good sleeping drug, too. That's why it's abused. My wife doesn't let me take it."

Dr. **James Oleske** arrived at UMDNJ as a medical student in 1968, never left and, eventually, rose to become professor of pediatrics. He has received a lifetime achievement award from the American Academy of Pediatrics for his work in children on the prevention, diagnosis and treatment of HIV/AIDs and in 2002 he was appointed medical director of the Circle of Life Foundation that is based here at the school.

Henry Leber Coit (1854-1917) was the first practicing pediatrician in Newark and in 1896 established the nation's second Babies' Hospital here. He is best known for calling attention to the dangers of impure milk and starting an international movement to "certify" that raw milk was produced by dairies under sanitary conditions regulated by a medical commission. Dr. Coit's method eventually was replaced by pasteurization, but he left his mark on pediatrics and public health far beyond his little hospital in Newark — and, long before Dr. Spock, he promoted education concerning how to care for healthy children and prevent disease.

Next was a long-time faculty member of the New Jersey Medical School, nephrologist **Richard Wedeen.** Starting in the early 1970s while working at the East Orange VA he focused on lead-induced hypertension and kidney disease. Dr. Wedeen helped to define the field of occupational renal diseases and has been a forceful advocate for lowering federal thresholds for safe lead levels in blood and water. His book *Poison in the Pot* (1984) reviewed the long history of lead poisoning and a later book *Toxic Circles* (1993) - co-edited with Helen Sheehan and with several other contributors - described other environmental health hazards such as mercury, chromium and dioxin all of which were prevalent in this heavily industrialized state.

Tied with Dr. Wedeen was someone who, I'm sure, few will recognize. **John B. Smith** (1858-1912) wasn't even a doctor. Born in 1858, he practiced law for five years before becoming fascinated by New Jersey's notorious mosquitos. I can't resist suggesting that he must have been bitten by the bug, or bugs - many times. Early settlers claimed that mosquitos caused more anguish than the "threat of Indians" and, during the 1880s when window screens were introduced, they were described as "the most humane contribution the 19th century made to the preservation of sanity and good temper." In addition to being annoying, mosquitos transmitted such scourges as malaria and yellow fever so when John B. Smith was appointed professor of entomology at Rutgers in 1889, he performed extensive research on the life cycles of mosquitos. Professor Smith produced more than 600 scientific and popular publications, including extensive catalogues of all the insects of New Jersey. He lobbied the legislature to fund various control projects in the salt marshes of the Meadowlands and along the Jersey shore which, happily, also turned out to be a boon to the tourist industry.

Fifth place was a tie between Drs. **Irving Selikoff** (1915-1992) and **Philip Levine** (1900-1987) with 9 votes each. Most everyone knows about Selikoff's documentation of asbestos-related diseases among workers at the Johns-Manville factory in Paterson. But probably few know that early in his career he was involved in research at Sea View Hospital on Staten Island that established the efficacy of isoniazid for treating TB — and for that work, he and his colleagues shared the prestigious Lasker Award for advances in medical research. When Irving Selikoff opened a general medicine practice in Paterson during the 1950s, he established a connection with the local Asbestos Workers Union and for the next thirty years, in hundreds of meetings and publications, he made both the profession and the public aware not only of the danger of asbestos, but of a deliberate cover-up by the asbestos industry. Industry fought back, demonized him and their vilification continued for a dozen years *after* Selikoff's death - an example of shooting the messenger long after he's left the scene! In his later years Irving Selikoff founded and directed the Environmental and Occupational Health Division of Mount Sinai Hospital that was named after him, and many have credited him with being the "Father" of the specialty of Occupational and Environmental Medicine.

Philip Levine was far less charismatic or controversial. He was an imuno-hematologist whose work advanced knowledge of the Rh factor, hemolytic disease of the newborn and blood transfusion. Born in Belarus in 1900, his family moved to this country when Levine was eight. He grew up in Brooklyn and in 1925, just two years out of Cornell Medical School, he became assistant to Nobel Laureate Karl Landsteiner at the Rockefeller

Institute. In 1935 Philip Levine became a bacteriologist at Newark's Beth Israel Hospital where, four years later, he and a colleague published a classic paper which suggested that a mother could make blood group antibodies as a result of immune sensitization to her fetus's red blood cells, and then pass them back to the fetus. At the time this was a common cause of maternal anemia and miscarriages and was responsible for the deaths of some 10,000 babies each year in this country. In 1946 (the second year it was given) the Lasker Award went to Dr. Levine along with his colleagues Karl Landsteiner and Alexander Wiener for their research in hematology.

In fourth place was Newark's own **Victor Parsonnet** (see Chapter 12) who pioneered the development of cardiac pacemakers and personally implanted many thousands — the last, I think, when he was age 87! He also led research on a nuclear pacemaker and an artificial heart and, among many other firsts, in 1986 he was the first New Jersey surgeon to perform a heart transplant.

Probably less well known to today's younger doctors was **Oscar Auerbach**, a pathologist who, while working at the East Orange VA during the 1960s, found the first evidence of a link between cancer and smoking in human lung tissue. Dr. Auerbach was a tireless investigator who sometimes examined 2,000 slides a day. He made careful clinical and pathological correlations and found that the more cigarettes were smoked, the greater the degree of tissue damage. When he trained dogs to smoke and studied the results, he refuted contentions by the tobacco industry that there was no cancer link. Dr. Auerbach wasn't a self promoter, just a dedicated investigator, respected by all, and his work provided the scientific basis for the Surgeon General's Report which in 1964 officially warned against the danger of smoking.

Prior to papers published by **Harrison Martland** (1883-1954) and his associates during the 1920s, radium was considered a boon to health, not a detriment. They described the clinical and pathological effects of radium poisoning in luminous watch dial painters in Orange, New Jersey who were continually pointing their brushes with their lips. Many of these young women had ingested radium and other chemicals and among the results was aplastic anemia (what he called "aregenerative" anemia) and certain bone tumors. Martland's documentation of radiation pathology helped implement safety standards and during World War II he consulted on protective devices for atomic workers. Dr. Martland served for 45 years as Newark's City Pathologist. He also was an authority on forensic medicine and it was he who coined the term "punch drunk." Maryland received international acclaim and numerous prestigious awards and several months before his death in 1954, Newark officials dedicated the Harrison S. Martland Medical Center across the street from here. (renamed in 1998 the Stanley S. Bergen Building.)

First place in our survey, with 19 of a possible 23 votes, went to the duo of **Selman Waksman** and his junior associate **Albert Schatz** for their discovery of streptomycin. Neither were physicians, but were soil biologists. The nature of their professional and personal relationships has been discussed frequently, perhaps best in Peter Pringle's book *Experiment Eleven.* In 1943 Schatz was a 23 year old graduate student working in Waksman's laboratory at Rutgers when he discovered streptomycin; indeed the younger man's name appeared first on their classic journal article and also was on the drug's patent application. Streptomycin was promoted as a "wonder drug more powerful than penicillin" and was the first effective antibiotic against tuberculosis.

However, controversy arose over whether Schatz was merely a junior member of a large team and to what extent his mentor deserved not only all the credit but the royalties as well. The dispute became nasty and was neither man's finest hour; the bottom line was the bottom line — money being the root of all evil. There were conflicting narratives and Schatz started a law suit. In 1950 a settlement was made between the two parties in which Schatz and several others shared in the profits, but two years later, when Selman Waksman was awarded the Nobel Prize, no mention was made of Schatz's contribution. Members of the medical establishment tended to favor Waksman's position as the Chief of the project. Schatz's subsequent career was rather undistinguished and some believe that he was blackballed as a troublemaker. Nevertheless, whoever was right or wrong, there's no question that the discovery of streptomycin was an enormous scientific advance and, as such, deserves recognition in our survey as perhaps New Jersey's most *important* medical event.

Or was it? I'm sure that my own choice for the New Jersey physician who had the greatest impact will come as a surprise. Earlier I mentioned Ezra Mundy Hunt who during the late 19th century was a leader in the public health movement. Another was Newark's Edgar Holden, the hero of Sandra Moss' recent book, who was instrumental in promoting large scale sewer construction to replace privies and cesspools. The work of pioneers like them was instrumental in combatting water borne infectious diseases.

However, the doctor whom I'd like to single out now probably won't be known to any of you. In fact his name didn't appear in our survey nor in any of the books that I've mentioned about New Jersey's medical history. I'd never heard of him until just last year when I watched a television program called *How We Got To Now* which discussed him (That show also appeared as a book with the same title written by Steven Johnson.)

Dr. **John L. Leal** (1858-1914) of Paterson, graduated from Princeton in 1880 and then obtained his medical degree from Columbia's College of Physicians and Surgeons. During the Civil War his physician father contracted amoebic dysentery from contaminated drinking water, eventually died from it and, no doubt, this influenced his son's career. Although he also treated patients, Dr. Leal had a passionate interest in public health, particularly concerning how to kill bacteria in public water supplies. He experimented with various techniques and in 1898 concluded that the most effective chemical was chlorine, then called calcium hypochlorite or chloride of lime. Previously it had been used as a disinfectant during outbreaks of typhoid and cholera but the characteristic smell of bleach was offensive and there was the crucial matter of correct dosage. Leal became convinced that if used in minute amounts, chlorine was the best way of killing germs without endangering humans. Eventually, he landed a job with the Jersey City Water Supply Company which gave him oversight of seven billion gallons of drinking water in the Passaic River watershed that supplied some 200,000 people.

This set the stage for one of the boldest interventions in the history of public health. There was a prolonged legal battle over contracts for reservoirs and water-supply pipes and Dr. Leal decided to put his experiments to the test. Working in almost complete secrecy and without first obtaining permission, he built a facility at the Boonton Reservoir which allowed the first mass chlorination of a city's water supply in history. Later Dr. Leal had to withstand scrutiny in two lengthy court hearings but his data was compelling and he testified that, in his opinion, Jersey City's water supply was the safest in the world. He prevailed and chlorination quickly became standard practice across the country and, eventually, all over. It's been estimated that the impact of chlorination, along with sand filtration and other methods of purifying drinking and bathing water, led to a 43% reduction in total mortality in the average American city and reduced infant and child mortality by more than 70% — and much of this was attributable to a mild-mannered New Jersey doctor who had the courage of his convictions. So, of all the people I've mentioned, he may have been the least famous but made the most long lasting contribution.

Probably New Jersey's most *famous* physician didn't even make our list because the question posed in our survey concerned what were the most *important* medical events in New Jersey's history and *not* who was the most famous doctor. **William Carlos Williams** of Rutherford was one of the greatest American poets but his medical work was mundane and certainly wouldn't qualify him for a Medical Hall of Fame according to our ground rules. "Doc" Williams, as his patients called him, was predominantly a pediatrician and served on the staffs of St. Mary's, Passaic General and Hackensack hospitals. While on house calls he often would stop his car by the roadside to scribble a few lines of verse on a blank prescription pad. William Carlos Williams published more than 3,000 poems, essays and stories and during the same four decade span, he delivered some 3,000 babies. He considered himself to be a man of the people, a doctor in the trenches, and had no use for medical politics or pomposity. Drawing inspiration from his humble working class patients, he once wrote that medicine and literature were "nearly the same thing...two parts of a whole."

No woman doctors made our list but, of course, there have been many outstanding individuals over the years. Perhaps the most well known was the anesthesiologist **Virginia Apgar** (1909-1974) who invented the so-called Apgar Scale which measures the health status of neonates. She grew up in Westfield and lived most of her life in Tenafly but mainly worked across the river at Columbia Presbyterian. Also there were many wonderful nurses from New Jersey including **Dorothea Dix** (1802-1881) the 19th century activist who lobbied throughout the country on behalf of the institutionalized mentally ill. Thanks to her, in 1848 New Jersey opened Trenton State Hospital, which was the most modern facility for care of the insane of its time, and during the Civil War she served as the Superintendent of Union Army Nurses. Speaking of army nurses, in 1901, during the Spanish-American War, while working with William Gorgas in Cuba, 24 year old **Clara Maas** (1876-1901) of East Orange volunteered to be bitten by mosquitos infected with yellow fever. After the first bite, she developed a mild case but when re-challenged to see whether she'd developed immunity, she hadn't — and died as a result. Two other volunteers also died and this put an end to yellow fever experiments on humans.

Karen Reeds suggested that I mention **Elizabeth Bugie,** a graduate student who worked in Selman Waksman's lab at Rutgers. Her name appeared on the landmark article in 1944 which announced the discovery of streptomycin, but wasn't on the follow-up article which described the drug's efficacy against TB, nor did it appear on the patent application. Many years later, she explained that she was told that because someday she'd get married and have a family, it wasn't important for her name to be on the patent. In 1952 after Albert Schatz successfully sued for his share of streptomycin's royalties, Waksman got 10%, Schatz 3% and two dozen others received token amounts - and among them was Elizabeth Bugie (Gregory) who received 0.2%. It amounted to only a few hundred dollars a year for the duration of the patent but it was a moral victory. I believe that she wound up becoming a librarian.

Medical historians like to celebrate our heroes and, I suppose, we all enjoy basking in their reflected glory. But New Jersey also has had its share of rogue doctors whose stories sometimes were more colorful than those of their conventional colleagues. Time permits me to only briefly mention a few candidates for my **Medical Hall of Shame** — like at Cooperstown, questions will arise about what qualifies or disqualifies someone for eligibility, but I'll let you judge that for yourselves. For example, we've had a few notorious murderers, probably including **Mario Jascalevitch** who during the 1960s gained fame as "Dr. X." He was chief of surgery at a small osteopathic hospital in Oradell and allegedly disposed of rival surgeons' postoperative patients by injecting them with curare. Events caught up with him nearly a decade after the actual deaths, but after many months of deliberation, a Grand Jury failed to find sufficiently clear and convincing evidence to convict him. Dr. X lost his license and fled back to his native Argentina, but his nickname persists in infamy. Less fortunate was the so-called "Angel of Death," male nurse **Charles Cullen** who confessed to killing up to 40 patients between 1988 and 2004 at at least five facilities. He didn't keep records and there've been estimates that he may have murdered as many as 400 people usually by injecting them with digoxin or insulin. Currently nurse Cullen is serving eleven consecutive life sentences totaling about 400 years!

New Jersey also has had its fair share of quacks and charlatans, my favorite being **Dinshah Ghadiali** (1873-1966) of Hillsdale and later Malaga. Born in Bombay, he claimed to have a dozen doctoral degrees including in engineering, law, chiropractic and "electro - hydrotherapy."

He said that he had one in medicine, too, but never produced a diploma. He certainly was versatile claiming to be an inventor, musician, linguist, mystic, yogi and pioneer aviator. When he arrived in Bergen County in 1911, he practiced his own unique form of medicine using what he called "spectochrome" therapy. It involved shining bright light passed through colored water in glass vials and aimed at the afflicted body part — naturally, he guaranteed marvelous results. Dinshah sold his projectors through the mails and for years battled the AMA and the US Postal Service. Although he spent two years in a Federal Penitentiary, that didn't stop him from running for Governor of New Jersey in 1925. Running from jail on a platform in which he asserted that he would promise nothing — he received more than 1000 votes!

In one of my books I described a man whom I dubbed "Dr. Evil." Dr. **Edwin Katzen-Ellenbogen** (1882-1955) was a German born psychiatrist who married an American and moved to her native city Boston. He became a naturalized American citizen, converted from Judaism to his wife's Catholicism and was an occasional lecturer at Harvard. He moved to New Jersey in 1911 where he worked for about two years at Skillman Village for Epileptics and then for another year at Trenton State Hospital. In 1914 he abandoned his family and returned to Europe where he developed a reputation as a bigamist, extortionist, forger and thief. During World War II the Nazis arrested him because of his Jewish roots and he was sent to Buchenwald where he collaborated with his captors. At trials after the war, other prisoners accused him of being responsible either directly or indirectly for the deaths of more than a thousand inmates. Although he claimed innocence, a U.S. Army tribunal at Dachau convicted him to a life sentence and he died in military prison. That's an unusual narrative for a Jewish born psychiatrist - a Harvard professor no less. It would seem that this psychopathologist was a psychopath.

When Katzen-Ellenbogen left Skillman for Trenton, his medical director there was Dr. **Henry Cotton** (1876-1933) about whom I've written before (see Chapter 3.) He wasn't really a villain — more a misguided megalomaniac who promoted the once popular idea that psychosis was due to focal infection with toxins traveling upstream from an occult source to the brain. The challenge was to find the offending pocket of pus and then to cut it out. Dr. Cotton claimed 85% success in curing psychosis and various other disorders with his knife. The NY Times praised him for what they described as "the most searching, aggressive and profound scientific investigation that has as yet been made in the whole field of mental and nervous disorders." The president of New Jersey's medical society declared that future generations "will rise up and call him blessed." Dr. Cotton's quest for occult focal infection would begin in the mouth where all of every patient's teeth were extracted. If that didn't work, next to go were the tonsils which started a national craze for prophylactic tonsillectomies. If mental symptoms still persisted, next various internal organs were removed - culminating with the large intestine. In 1919 alone, Dr. Cotton ordered more than 6000 dental extractions, more than 500 tonsillectomies and 79 total colectomies on his mental patients. Although the colectomies had a mortality of between 30 and 40%, he insisted that these were desperate end-stage cases - it was their last chance. Alas, it was all too good to be true. Inevitably, there were investigations; his results couldn't be replicated and Henry Cotton's crusade against pus ended in 1933 when he suddenly died from a heart attack. Nevertheless, tonsils continued to be removed everywhere — including my own — as prevention against whatever.

Finally, I'd be remiss if I didn't state the obvious - that the vast majority of The Garden State's physicians neither qualified for an honorary Hall of Fame nor a Hall of Shame. They worked diligently, honorably and usually without acclaim and it is those often under-appreciated colleagues whom we really should celebrate. So let's raise a *virtual* toast to our predecessors who have served New Jersey so well and for so long.

17. CHAIRMAN MAO'S WESTERN DOCTORS

My interest in this subject evolved over time as a result of three personal experiences which I'll explain along the way. But I'll begin by describing two remarkable doctors about whom, at first, I knew nothing.

George Hatem was born in 1910 into a poor Lebanese-American family in Buffalo, NY. He grew up and was educated in North Carolina, studied medicine first in Beirut and then obtained his degree in Geneva, Switzerland. In 1933, along with two classmates, Lazar Katz and Robert Levinson, he sailed for China. All of them were passionate about helping the needy and faced with the choice either to fight fascism in Spain or sail for China to fight poverty and venereal disease, they chose the latter.

The three young doctors opened a practice in Shanghai which prospered largely by treating the diseases of foreign prostitutes. Soliciting support from wealthy members of the large expatriate Jewish community there, his friends encouraged Hatem to say that he was a Sephardic Jew. Indeed, although he was a Maronite Christian, Hatem often was mistaken for being Jewish and, like his two companions, had experienced discrimination and poverty. After three years George's partners, disenchanted by Shanghai's corruption and poverty, returned home but he remained and having become supportive of the communist cause, declared that he wanted to be "a revolutionary doctor." By 1936 Mao had begun his Long March to the mountains of Northwest China and sent out a message that he needed "an honest journalist and a doctor." As George Hatem later joked, "they didn't ask for an honest doctor so they took me." The journalist turned out to be Edgar Snow who later recalled things differently, quoting Hatem: "I didn't spend my old man's money learning to be a VD quack for a gangster society. Maybe these people up north are interested in putting an end to the whole business. I want to see what they're like."

The two travelled extensively throughout rural China, but although Snow soon would become world famous for writing about what he saw in his book *Red Star Over China,* Dr. Hatem asked that his name not be mentioned in Snow's reports. In fact, the twenty-eight year old doctor kept such a low profile that his family didn't know whether he even was alive for nearly five decades!

George Hatem was not a Communist and at first spoke no Chinese, but he was blessed with a congenial personality and quickly gained the respect of Mao and his staff in their mountain enclave. There had been a rumor that Mao was gravely ill or dead but The Chairman permitted Hatem to examine him and he was found to be in good health. That was important because a foreign doctor's testimony could be trusted. Hatem assumed the name Ma Hai-teh (Ma means horse; Hai-teh loosely translated, "virtue from overseas".) He was familiarly known as Dr. Ma ("Dr. Horse") and received no money for his work; only a special meat ration. Later I will return to George Hatem's story but it seems that he was able to convince Mao of a critical need to attract well-trained foreign doctors and, as it happened, there was an available pool of willing candidates in France.

When the Spanish Civil War broke out in 1936 hundreds of doctors from all over the world volunteered to join the so-called International Brigade - the American contingent was known as The Abraham Lincoln Brigade and 59 of 124 doctors were Jewish. After Franco's forces defeated the Spanish Loyalists in 1939, many doctors returned home but some crossed the Pyrenees into France where they were detained in squalid internment camps. A British and Norwegian committee asked for volunteers for the International Red Cross's Medical Relief Corp (IRMC) in China, which had been invaded by Japan two years earlier, and twenty of the internees were selected out of fifty applicants. When the largest of three contingents arrived in China on October 16,1939, the Chinese called them "Spanish Doctors" although none were Spaniards; four came from Poland, three each from Germany and Austria and ten from eight other countries. More than half were Jewish, including the Poles (Stanislaw Flato, Leon Kamieniecki, Wolf Jungerman and Victor Taubenfligel), Bulgarian Janto Kaneti and Austrian Fritz Jensen. They lived under the same primitive conditions as the troops, received no pay and asked only to be sent to the front lines where they could apply the lessons they'd learned in Spain.

The first doctor to arrive from Spain (alone and of his own volition) was Norman Bethune, a 48 year old Canadian thoracic surgeon. A melodramatic biography *The Scalpel, the Sword* written by journalists Ted Allan and Sydney Gordon was published in 1952 with a preface by Madame Sun Yat-Sen. The book contained long passages from the doctor's diary, appeared in nineteen languages and sold more than a million copies. Bethune's life story resembled a Hollywood movie - especially as embellished by his enthusiastic biographers.

Norman Bethune was born in Ontario in 1890, grew up there and when Canada entered World War I, while still a medical student he was among the first to enlist. For nearly a year he served as a stretcher-bearer in France until he was seriously wounded by shrapnel and sent home to recover. During this time he received his medical degree in 1916 and promptly rejoined the military - first the Royal Navy and then transferring to the Flying Corps. After the war Bethune had a small general surgical practice in Detroit, but was depressed with his marriage and unhappy with social and economic conditions. Moody, irritable, impatient, obsessed by work, he led a sybaritic and unorthodox life style and drank to excess.

Then in 1924, at age 34, he developed severe pulmonary TB. Expecting to die soon, he insisted that his wife divorce him so she'd be free to lead her own life. Unburdened from responsibility for her, he entered Trudeau's famous sanitorium in Saranac Lake and prepared for the inevitable. However it didn't come as quickly as expected and after about two years there, while at lowest ebb, he read in a medical journal about a new technique of lung compression that promised a second chance of life for him. Having nothing to lose, he underwent several pneumothorax procedures and made a miraculous recovery. After discharge from Trudeau's sanitorium Bethune remarried his former wife (later she divorced him a second time) and dedicated himself to becoming a thoracic surgeon. Studying with one of Canada's leading chest surgeons he became a prominent figure in Montreal and developed a fine reputation as a proponent of lung compression. He performed thousands of thoracoplastys, invented more than a dozen types of surgical instruments, published his findings in medical journals and became an outspoken crusader against TB which he insisted could be conquered if only enough resources were provided to fight "The White Plague.".

In varying degrees, Norman Bethune also was a poet, painter, art collector and political theorist. By turns, arrogant or compassionate, ascetic or hedonistic, he spent lavishly and recklessly and, although he became a wealthy society doctor, gave freely of his services and money to the poor. During this period he was increasingly troubled by the failure of organized medicine to address inequities in health care during the Great Depression. Scorning hypocrisy in the medical profession and injustice in society, he was attracted to radical political ideas and became a vocal advocate for socialized medicine. After an extended observational visit to Russia in 1935, he joined the communist party and the next year left for Spain to fight fascism. Observing the slaughter first-hand, often at great danger to himself, he organized mobile medical and blood transfusion units to treat wounded troops on front-lines that stretched more than a thousand miles. In 1937 he returned to Canada to raise money to fight the fascists in Spain and spoke to as many as 15,000 people at a time throughout North America.

However the Spanish Civil War was going badly for the Loyalists and when Bethune learned that China had been invaded by the Japanese, he decided to leave home again. In a letter to his ex-wife he wrote, "I refuse to live in a world that spawns murder and corruption without raising my hand against them. I refuse to condone, by passivity or by default, the wars which greedy men make against others.... Spain and China are part of the same battle. I am going to China because I feel this is where the need is greatest; that is where I can be most useful..."

When Norman Bethune arrived in 1938, he travelled many hundreds of miles on horseback to find Mao at his enclave in the north. Upon arrival he was warmly *greeted by Dr. Ma (George Hatem)* who explained the critical need for an experienced surgeon of the Canadian's ability. During their several hour meeting, Bethune and Mao developed mutual respect. Bethune was surprised by Mao's erudition and wrote, "The man is a giant. He is one of the great men of the world." Mao listened carefully as Bethune described his experiences in Spain and, in particular, was impressed by his claim that 75 percent of serious battle casualties could be saved if they were treated right at the front. Mao commissioned Bethune to organize a mobile medical unit and for the next nearly two years his slogan, which was adapted by his followers, was "Doctors! Go to the wounded! Do not wait for them to come to you." Tall and bearded, Norman Bethune made a striking figure on horseback. The locals were in awe of the stamina and skill of the man they called Pai Chu En (white-seek-grace.) Once he performed seventy operations in 40 hours with only one death; another time 115 operations in 69 hours. Mules transported the equipment, including a mobile blood bank, hundreds of miles over rough mountain trails in extreme weather conditions. Bethune convinced frightened villagers to donate blood which was stored in cold streams along the route.

Dr. Bethune set up mobile hospitals in caves and abandoned Buddhist temples. He regularly reported back to Mao who appointed him medical chief of the 8th Route Army and adviser to the entire region. His assistants and nurses were uneducated peasants who made up in enthusiasm and courage for what they lacked in training. He scheduled educational programs and as they sat at his feet on mud floors, he lectured on anatomy, physiology and wound care. He wrote a medical handbook and established a training school to provide a continuing supply of capable medical workers in the future. Bethune wrote in his diary that it took "a combination of shouts, tears and smiles to get things done.... I have come to love them; I know they love me too." Although the Chinese were determined to provide him with a token salary of $100 a month, he refused, asking them to spend the money on cigarettes and food for the starving troops.

During Norman Bethune's time in China Dr. Ma served as his liaison both to Mao's command group and also with the outside world. He sometimes sent magazines and newspapers but Bethune received only five letters from home the whole time. When he had a spare moment he was lonely and toward the end he wrote, "I sometimes dream of coffee, rare roast beef, of apple pie and ice cream. Mirages of heavenly food. Books... Are books still being written? Is music still being played? Do you dance, drink beer, look at pictures? What do clean sheets feel like in a soft bed? Do women still love to be loved?" Then in November, 1939, under fire from nearby Japanese troops, he cut his finger while operating without gloves. He considered the wound to be trivial but without antibiotics it festered and within a few days he was dead at age 49. The heart-broken troop's battle cry had been "Attack! Bethune is with us!" Now it became "Remember Dr. Bethune!"

Although hardly known in his native Canada, Norman Bethune's legend grew in China until he achieved iconic status. Chairman Mao's eulogy, which was memorized by generations of young people, concluded with these words: "Dr. Bethune's devotion to the common people is a lesson for us all. The manner in which we commemorate his death indicates how deep an imprint his personality has made on us. All of us should emulate his unselfish spirit. It should become a starting point for us to become individuals useful to the people. An individual may have great or little ability, but with such a spirit he can become a man of importance, of integrity, of virtue who forsakes self-interest for the interest of the people." Hospitals and a medical school were named for him, statues erected in many places and, to this day, throngs regularly visit Dr. Bethune's grave and mausoleum.

My interest in this subject began nearly twenty years ago when my wife and I took three tourist trips respectively to China, Japan and India that were led by Rabbi Marvin Tokayer. During the 1960s he had served as a U.S. Air Force chaplain based in Japan and later returned and worked for eight years as rabbi for the small Jewish community living in Japan. In this capacity he became an authority on all things Jewish in the Far East and it was on one of Rabbi Tokayer's popular trips, "China Through Jewish Eyes," that I first learned from him about a Viennese urologist by the name of Jakob Rosenfeld. In 1939, denied escape from Nazi Germany to the West, he fled eastward to China which by then was under Japanese control. Indeed his story is quite as dramatic as those of Drs. Bethune and Hatem.

Jakob Rosenfeld (1903-1952) was born in Lemberg (Lvov) into a prosperous assimilated Jewish family. His family moved to Vienna where he graduated from medical school in 1928. He trained as a urologist and shared a private practice with his sister, but when the Nazis marched into Austria in March 1938 he was arrested by the Gestapo as an outspoken anti-Fascist and liberal intellectual. He was sent to Dachau and then transferred to Buchenwald where he covertly treated patients and performed illegal operations. After more than a year he was released with the proviso that he leave Austria within fourteen days. It was impossible to obtain a visa in such a short time but he was able to secure passage on a ship bound for Shanghai where some 25,000 European Jews were accepted without visas. Once arrived Dr. Rosenfeld opened a urology practice in the neighborhood called "Little Vienna" and befriended a group of Austrian ex-patriots who were sympathetic to the Chinese Communist party. He condemned America for supplying war materials to the Japanese in order to arm them against the Russians - it was prior to Pearl Harbor. Appalled by the abject poverty of the Chinese population and their desperate health conditions, he decided to help. In early 1941, when he offered his service to Mao's army, he was warned of the hard life that he would face; Rosenfeld replied that if he could survive Buchenwald he would do fine. And when he travelled through enemy lines to reach the 4th New Army's headquarters, the doctor joined the troops in chanting, "Down with Fascism! Down with Hitler! Down with Chiang Kai-shek!"

Jakob Rosenfeld served in the army for eight years and in his memoirs, which were published many years later, he described how he established clinics, instructed medical staff in fundamentals of hygiene and sanitation and treated soldiers and civilians for malaria, typhus, dysentery, scabies, anemia and malnutrition. He was appointed Commander of the Medical Corps of the People's Liberation Army, equivalent to the rank of general - indeed he often was called "General Luo." He provided medical care to several elite officers who later would become leaders of the Communist government, but after the war ended Jakob Rosenfeld developed heart trouble and realized the need for specialized treatment.

In 1949 Dr. Rosenfeld returned to Vienna for medical care but no longer felt at home there and was unwilling to seek hospital work with former Nazis as colleagues. In an epilogue to his memoirs (1950) he vilified America and lauded Communist China: "The Idols are dead. Japan, Chiang Kai-shek and Wall Street no longer matter. Long life to the New China!" But Mao's xenophobic government refused him permission to reenter - their reason remains controversial; perhaps it was more a bureaucratic slip-up than by design, but feeling betrayed Rosenfeld now found himself to be a man without a country. Refused a visa to the United States because of his Communist ties, he sought respite in Switzerland and then asylum in the recently established state of Israel. He arrived in 1951 there and for nearly two years worked at Assuta Hospital in Tel Aviv before dying of a sudden heart attack in April, 1952. Many years later, Jakob Rosenfeld was remembered in exhibitions held in Vienna and Tel Aviv and in China a memorial statue was erected and a research center and a hospital were named after the man whom they once nicknamed "The Buddha's Savior."

At about the same time that I first wrote about Jakob Rosenfeld in one of my books *Jewish Medical Roots* (published in 2003) another author, Frank Heynick, published a massive book titled *Jews and Medicine* that contained a surprising statement:

> *Mao tae-tung would have a Jewish physician, yet this was not a Chinese but a Soviet Jew (who, incidentally, was arrested on Stalin's orders for supposedly being involved in the so-called Doctors' Plot.)*

I wondered whether Heynick might be referring to Jakob Rosenfeld and decided to investigate. (I won't discuss that subject in depth here; in fact, my conclusions were published in 2004 in *Korot*, a Jewish medical history journal published in Israel.) But my title asked the question, "Did Chairman Mao Have a Jewish Doctor?" and after reviewing the author's sources and considering potential candidates, I concluded that he did not. Concerning Jakob Rosenfeld, I found no evidence that he ever met Chairman Mao whom he greatly admired. To be sure, Rosenfeld dedicated his diary to "The Genius of the new China" and in 1948 he had joined hundreds of others on a triumphant march to Beijing where he heard Mao proclaim the People's Republic and command "Complete the Revolution." Dr. Rosenfeld considered this to be the high point of his life and in his memoirs compared Mao's Long March to refuge in the mountains to Moses leading the Israelites through the desert.

Well if not Jakob Rosenfeld, could Frank Heynick have meant George Hatem/Dr. Ma? In his role as general medical adviser, it's conceivable that he might have had occasion to give personal medical advice to the Chairman. Indeed, in his autobiography (see later) Dr. Li Zhisui quoted Mao as saying, "Dr. George Hatem came and stayed with us for good and has made great contributions to our campaign to eliminate venereal disease." However, because Hatem never served as Mao's personal physician, when my article was published in *Korot* in 2004, I concluded:

> *Fifty years after Stalin's Doctors' Plot, the trail of Mao's alleged Jewish doctor has grown cold and there is no reliable evidence that any foreign physician - Russian, Jewish or otherwise - had access to Chairman Mao during the early 1950s."*

I thought that would be my last word about this material, but a dozen years later in May 2016 the subject came up again when I met Professor Andrzej Krakowski who as a young man in 1968 was exiled from his native Poland along with some 20,000 other Jews. In the United States he went on to become an acclaimed Hollywood movie director and producer and for many years has taught film and video arts at the City University of New York. To my great surprise, Professor Krakowski told me that when he was a boy growing up in Warsaw he met a close friend of his parents who was a Jewish doctor who had treated Chairman Mao. Considering what I'd written a dozen years earlier, I was skeptical about the last part but was eager to learn more.

Stanislaw (Szmul Mosze) Flato, was born in Warsaw in 1910 into a wealthy Jewish merchant family. While a medical student in Paris the left-leaning and idealistic young man joined the communist party and after graduation in 1936 he volunteered for the International Brigade in Spain and soon rose to rank of major and headed the medical service of the 35th Division. After the Fascist's victory, he was kept in a French internment camp for nearly a year until in the summer of 1939 he was among the twenty medical volunteers who agreed to work for the International Red Cross in China; in fact he headed one of the contingents, participated in several daring rescue missions and organized a field medical school to train the raw medical personnel. The Chinese called him Fu Lato (later Fu Ladu) and, as Professor Krakowski explained, he became "the personal physician and a confident of Chairman Mao and the elite of the Chinese leaders." In 1942 Major Flato was one of nine "Spanish Doctors" who were "loaned" to General Joseph ("Vinegar Joe") Stilwell's unit then operating in the jungles of Burma and remained there for twenty months. After the end of World War II eight of the "Spanish Doctors" remained for a while in China working for the United Nations Relief and Rehabilitation Association (UNRRA) but right after the war, in September 1945, Flato returned to Poland for the first time in fifteen years. He served in several capacities, including as a colonel on the military staff from 1946 to 1952, but his fortunes changed in 1953 during a purge of former members of the International Brigade who were politically suspect. He was falsely accused of being a CIA agent, imprisoned and tortured by the hard-line Polish regime. But when his former Chinese colleagues learned of his situation, Chou En lai was sent on a diplomatic visit to Warsaw and intervened to save him.

After he was "rehabilitated," Dr. Flato was named as the first Polish ambassador to the People's Republic of China. Returning to Beijing in 1957 as Chief Adviser for the Polish Embassy, he remained there until 1964 when he returned to Poland and worked in the Ministry of Foreign Affairs. However, during the Polish government's anti-Semitic purges of March 1968, he was removed from his government position and, unlike many thousand of other Jews, he was not permitted to emigrate because he knew too much about military and foreign affairs. In 1972 while on a family trip to East Berlin Stanislaw Flato died suddenly at age 62.

In June 2016 Xi Jinping, President of The People's Republic of China, spoke in Warsaw about the two country's mutual friendship during World War II and specifically cited Stanislaw Flato as one of many Poles who had provided support for the embattled Chinese during their war against Japan. Four months later, Professor Krakowski lectured about Dr. Flato in Shanghai and much of what I've described here is based on his work.

Did any of this new information about Dr. Flato and the other "Spanish Doctors" help answer my question, "Did Chairman Mao Have a Jewish Doctor?" I think not. Frank Heynick's statement in his book *Jews and Medicine* read, "Mao tae-tung would have a Jewish physician, yet this was not a Chinese but a Soviet Jew (who, incidentally was arrested on Stalin's orders for supposedly being involved in the so-called Doctor's Plot." The word "would" might mean that Mao *did* have a Jewish doctor or perhaps that he *wanted* one - if the former, did that mean for his personal doctor. or merely as a member of his staff? Half of the "Spanish Doctors" working with the Chinese army were Jewish - including Stanislaw Flato - and there were a very few others as well. (For example, in 1946-7 a German Jewish dentist Magdalene Robitscher-Hahn treated him on ten occasions for gum disease and filled several cavities.)

Nevertheless, Heynick's statement about Mao having a Russian Jewish doctor who later was arrested and prosecuted in Stalin's infamous Doctor's Plot of 1953 seems totally implausible. It is true that many of the prominent doctors who were falsely accused of plotting to murder Russian leaders were Jewish, but whether any of them had access to Mao is doubtful. When a Chinese delegation headed by The Chairman travelled to Moscow in 1949 to attend the 40th Anniversary celebration of the October Revolution, the Russians assigned a doctor to be at Mao's beck and call, but having little to do, apparently he spent most of his time drinking vodka and then sleeping it off. In any case, none of the physicians discussed here were Russian and only Drs. Rosenfeld and Flato were Jewish. To be sure, Dr. Hatem sometimes was mistakenly thought to be Jewish - once a Russian agent reported to Moscow that he was "Jewish by nationality [and] a citizen of New Zealand."

From the early 1930s and for the next two decades the chief physician for Mao and other communist leaders was Fu Lianzhang (aka Nelson Fu.) Baptized as a Christian and trained at a Christian medical school, he was known as "the Christian doctor" and had participated in the Long March. But Fu was a political schemer and fell out of favor with Mao (he was tortured to death during the Cultural Revolution in 1968.) After the new government was formed in 1949, each leader was assigned a personal physician. Dr. Xu Tao was Mao's first until in 1954 he was assigned to become Mao's demanding wife Jiang Qing's physician. There were a few others until In 1955 thirty-five year old Dr. Li Zhisui reluctantly took over what soon became his full-time job - for the next twenty-two years! Serving both as medical adviser and confidant, he was almost constantly at the leader's side and, in effect, the isolated Chairman's only friend. Dr. Li had been well trained in the Rockefeller Foundation sponsored Peking Union Medical College and initially was assigned to head the health clinic at the compound where Mao and other leaders resided. Although he revered Mao as a great leader, familiarity gradually led to contempt, but out of fear of his own and his family's safety he never felt able to resign. It wasn't until 1988, a dozen years after Mao's death, that he and his wife finally were able to join their family in the United States where he began writing his memoir, *The Private Life of Chairman Mao* (Random House, 1954.) There was much to say and the tell-all book was 649 pages long. Shortly after the book appeared, Dr. Li died suddenly at his home in Chicago. The official cause was a heart attack but some suspected that he had been poisoned.

In his memoir Dr. Li described Mao as a medically unsophisticated person who had an aversion for all physicians and frequently advised others to follow only half of what was prescribed. Dr. Li wrote that in 1951 "a team of Soviet physicians had examined him, poking and prodding for so long that Mao lost his temper." But from 1955 on the paranoid Chairman insisted that no one other than his personal doctor be permitted to attend him. Being in such close proximity, Dr. Li was subject to suspicion by sycophants and intriguers in the Byzantine-like court. It was not unusual for him to have to sample Mao's medicine and more than once he was accused by Mao's scheming wife of attempting to poison both of them. As a virtual prisoner Dr. Li had to share the Chairman's eccentric and insomniac life-style. Mao did not bathe or brush his teeth, preferring to rinse his mouth with tea which blackened his teeth. He didn't dress for days at a time preferring to lounge nearly naked beside his private swimming pool amidst a bevy of young peasant women. According to Dr. Li, among Mao's predilections was a fondness for young women and until his final years the Chairman was surrounded by a virtual harem of comely women. He identified with the legendary first Chinese emperor, known as "The Yellow Emperor," who was reported to have become immortal by making love to a thousand virgins; Mao believed that the more sexual liaisons he had, the longer he would live and there was no lack of willing partners. As he aged, on occasion Mao couldn't perform and agreed to take daily injections of "formula Vitamin E3 (Novocaine) prescribed by a Rumanian woman Dr. Lepshinskaya. Dr. Li administered the injections - after first taking them himself to ensure safety - but alas, there was no aphrodisiac effect and after three months the regimen was discontinued. In his last years Mao suffered from complications of amyotrophic lateral sclerosis and heart and lung failure and in 1976 after a series of heart attacks the Chairman died at age 82.

What became of George Hatem/"Dr. Ma"? In 1960, after a twenty-five year absence, Edgar Snow returned to China and described his trip in magazine articles and another massive book, *The Other Side of the River.* Recalling how he met his old friend "Dr. Horse" again, this time Snow devoted two chapters to the man whom he described as a medical "missionary" - the only western doctor who volunteered for service "on the other side of the river." In the interim, "Dr. Horse" had married a beautiful Chinese actress and they had two children - their names translated as "Second Horse" and "Little Pony." Edgar Snow preferred using the nickname "Shag" for his friend which apparently referred to his hirsute appearance in younger days. Once in a serious moment, Shag explained why he had left his successful practice in Shanghai a quarter century earlier:

> *I don't give a damn for a doctor who lives high by pampering the neurotic rich. The medical profession is a failure if we can't give all children of even the humblest parentage an equal start in life - the same food and proper care that only the wealthy can afford now. If that's what these people up there are aiming at, I'm with them...*

George Hatem served the medical needs of Mao's army for a decade and after the Communists took control in 1949, he was the first foreigner to be granted citizenship in the People's Republic. He always tried to integrate western and traditional Chinese medicine (Mao approved) and emphasized hygiene and preventive public health efforts. After the war ended teams led by Dr Hatem, known as "Chairman Mao's Doctors," were sent into desolate areas where they eliminated the ancient scourge of leprosy. Although he did his best to distance himself from political intrigue, as a foreigner Hatem's motives were suspect and, despite his reputation as the most loved American in China, during the Cultural Revolution he was denounced as a "bourgeois lackey." Worse, he was accused of being an American spy and only late in life was permitted to travel outside.

By the time that Edgar Snow and George Hatem resumed their friendship in 1960, "Shag" was fifty years old and chief of staff of an Institute of Venereology and Skin Diseases with a staff of about six hundred. He explained in great detail how the campaigns against venereal disease and leprosy had been conducted. In his second book Snow noted that for a quarter century Hatem had been the only American who intimately shared the ordeals of the people who fought to bring China to her feet. He knew the faults and failures of the regime but also knew the misery of Old China and the enormity of the problems it presented. He asked Edgar Snow to tell his family in America that he was "a very lucky and happy man." At the same time he couldn't understand how his friend could be happy in a "still unredeemed society":

> *Repeatedly [Hatem] expressed the warmest and sincerest kind of concern for his fellow countrymen in America, who had yet to begin the ascent toward an enlightened civilization and objectives such as he obviously fully approved of, in China....'China simply could never have stood up in any other way. Nearly everything done has been necessary and nearly everything necessary has been done. And all in all it's a success.'*

In 1986, two decades after his reunion with Edgar Snow, George Hatem finally returned to the United States to receive the prestigious Albert Lasker Public Service Award in recognition of his work in virtually saving millions of Chinese lives. The official citation said in part: "Dr. Ma's contributions can be compared in importance to the eradication of yellow fever and the bubonic plague, and as a model for the public health control of venereal diseases, they stand alone." While in the United States to receive the award, in a lengthy interview (which can be viewed on-line) he proved to be a thoughtful and eloquent analyst when speculating about how principles of prevention that had worked in China might be applied in this country which then was experiencing the first AIDS epidemic. Two years later George Hatem died of cancer at age 78 in Beijing.

Although Drs. Hatem and Flato certainly had direct access to The Chairman, it seems unlikely that any of the four doctors described here provided significant personal care to Mao Tse-tung either during the war years or afterward. Because of their political views Drs. Bethune and Rosenfeld were pariahs in the West and today their names are hardly known here. Nevertheless, millions of Chinese revered these Western doctors for their profound contributions to public health - and they still do.

www.ingramcontent.com/pod-product-compliance
Lightning Source LLC
Chambersburg PA
CBHW030949180526
45163CB00002B/715